Prescription for Nutritional Healing

The A-to-Z Guide to Supplements

Prescription for Nutritional Healing

The A-to-Z Guide to Supplements

2ND EDITION

Based on Part One of *Prescription for Nutritional Healing,* Third Edition

PHYLLIS A. BALCH, CNC

AVERY

a member of Penguin Putnam Inc.

New York

Every effort has been made to ensure that the information contained in this book is complete and accurate. However, neither the publisher nor the author is engaged in rendering professional advice or services to the individual reader. The ideas, procedures, and suggestions contained in this book are not intended as a substitute for consulting with your physician. All matters regarding health require medical supervision. Neither the author nor the publisher shall be liable for any loss, injury, or damage allegedly arising from any information or suggestion in this book.

Most Avery books are available at special quantity discounts for bulk purchase for sales promotions, premiums, fund-raising, and educational needs. Special books or book excerpts also can be created to fit specific needs. For details, write Putnam Special Markets, 375 Hudson Street, New York, NY 10014.

a member of
Penguin Putnam Inc.
375 Hudson Street
New York, NY 10014
www.penguinputnam.com

Library of Congress Cataloging-in-Publication Data

Balch, Phyllis A., date.
Prescription for nutritional healing : the A to Z guide to supplements /
Phyllis A. Balch, James F. Balch.—2nd ed.
p. cm.
Includes index.
ISBN 1-58333-143-3
1. Nutrition—Popular works. 2. Dietary supplements—Popular works.
3. Herbs—Therapeutic use—Popular works. I. Title.
RA784.B2483 2002   2002016433
613.2—dc21

Printed in the United States of America
3 5 7 9 10 8 6 4 2

Book design by Tanya Maiboroda

CONTENTS

PREFACE

*"A wise man should consider that health is
the greatest of human blessings."*
—Hippocrates

Socrates once said, "There is only one good, knowledge, and one evil, ignorance." This statement should guide us in all of our actions, especially where our health is concerned. Too many of us do not have the slightest idea of how to maintain good health. When illness strikes, we rely on our doctors to cure us. What we fail to realize is that "the cure" comes from within. Nature has provided us with a wondrous immune system, and all we have to do is take proper care of this inner healing force.

Does this sound too simple? Basically, it is simple; our modern lifestyles have gotten us off the right track, with fast foods, alcohol abuse, drug dependencies, a polluted environment, and high-tech stress. Nature intended to fuel our inner healing force with the right natural substances to enable the body to function up to its fullest potential. Nature's resources—whole foods, vitamins, minerals, enzymes, amino acids, phytochemicals, and other natural bounties—are designed for use in our immune systems. However, because most of us have a profound lack of knowledge as to what our bodies need to function properly, we find ourselves out of balance and susceptible to all sorts of illnesses.

All individuals should take an active part in the maintenance of their health and in the treatment of their disorders with the guidance of a health care professional. The more we take it upon ourselves to learn about nutrition, the better prepared we will be to take that active role. Attitude is also an important factor in the processes of health maintenance and healing. We must have a positive state of mind in order to bring harmony to the body. The realization that body (lifestyle), spirit (desire), and mind (belief) must come together is the first step to better health.

This new edition has taken over twenty-five years of study, work, and research to put together. It is intended to provide you and your health care professional with a more natural approach to healing, which may be used in conjunction with your current medical treatment. A number of the suggestions offered, such as intravenous therapy, can be administered only by or under the supervision of a licensed physician. Also, because our body chemistries differ, some of us may have allergic reactions to certain supplements. Before taking any nutritional supplement, check with your health care professional regarding its appropriateness. Should you experience an allergic reaction to any supplement, immediately discontinue use of the supplement. You should never attempt to treat yourself without professional advice.

No statement in this publication should be construed as a claim for cure, treatment, or prevention of any disease. It is also important to point out that you should not reject mainstream medical methods. Learn about your condition, and don't be afraid to ask questions. Feel free to get second and even third opinions from qualified health professionals. It is a sign of wisdom, not cowardice, to seek more knowledge through your active participation as a patient.

Every effort has been made to include the latest research available on nutritional healing. We also have added new sections on many health disorders at the suggestions of our readers. All the information in this book has been carefully researched, and the data have been reviewed and updated throughout the production process. Because this body of knowledge promises to continue growing and changing, we suggest that when questions arise, you refer to other current sources of information to verify textual material. We will strive to keep abreast of new scientific information, treatments, and supplements, and make this information available to you in future editions of this book.

Over 800 years ago, Moses Maimonides said, "The physician should not treat the ailment, but the patient who is suffering from it." This book was designed to meet the differing needs of individuals and to help each person create his or her own nutritional program.

ABOUT THIS BOOK

WE HAVE LEARNED a great deal from traveling the country and speaking to so many of the people who have used our book *Prescription for Nutritional Healing*. That book was designed to be a comprehensive in-home guide that would help you to achieve and maintain the highest possible level of health and fitness through careful dietary planning and nutritional supplementation. However, we found we were frequently asked whether we could design a book that would provide basic information on a wide variety of today's nutritional supplements, and yet easily fit into a pocket or handbag to be taken to the store, on trips, or wherever needed—an edition that would incorporate up-to-date findings in the fields of nutrition and supplementation, from old standbys like vitamin C to newer products such as cordyceps, SAMe, and olive leaf extract. The answer to this question is *Prescription for Nutritional Healing: The A-to-Z Guide to Supplements*. Now in its second edition, this book was specifically created to provide on-the-go readers with authoritative information drawn from Part One of *Prescription for Nutritional Healing*, packaged in a handy reference that you can take along with you wherever you go. This volume provides all the information needed to design your own personal nutritional program as well as to use and understand today's supplements. What you will find here is a clear discussion of the basic principles of nutrition and health, as well as lists and explanations of the various types of nutrients, food supplements, and herbs found in health food shops and drugstores. Topics covered include vitamins, minerals, water, amino acids, antioxidants, enzymes, a wide variety of natural food supplements, and herbs.

Before you start any supplement regimen on a regular basis, test the supplements one at a time to find out if you have a reaction to any of them. Always listen to your body. If you experience unpleasant effects you suspect may be linked to a particular supplement, either discontinue the supplement or decrease the dosage.

Always take supplements with a full glass of water. Nutritional supplements are concentrated and can overburden the liver if you do not consume sufficient liquid with them. In addition, water enhances absorption and is needed to aid in carrying the nutrients to the cells.

If you follow a nutritional supplementation program for longer than a year, change brands periodically so that you do not develop an intolerance or build up a resistance to one or more of the ingredients in any given supplement. Remember, you can develop an intolerance to the ingredients in vitamins and other supplements just as you can to foods.

It is important for us to stress that the information offered in this book is not intended to replace appropriate medical advice and prescribed treatment. The use of any of the supplements recommended here should be approved and monitored by your medical doctor or other trained health-care professional.

INTRODUCTION

THE BODY IS a complex organism that has the ability to heal itself—if only you listen to it and respond with proper nourishment and care. In spite of all the abuse our bodies endure—whether through exposure to environmental toxins, poor nutrition, cigarette smoking, alcohol consumption, or inactivity—they still usually serve us well for many years before signs of illness may start to appear. Even then, with a little help, they respond and continue to function.

The human body is the greatest machine on earth. Nerve signals travel through muscles at speeds as fast as 200 miles per hour. The brain puts out enough electric power to light a 20-watt light bulb. If your leg muscles moved as fast as your eye muscles, you could walk over fifty miles in one day. According to scientists, bone is among the strongest building materials known to humankind; it can withstand nearly as much stretching and bending stress as, and more compression stress than, steel-reinforced concrete can tolerate.

Think of your body as being composed of millions of tiny little engines. Some of these engines work in unison; some work independently. All are on call twenty-four hours a day. In order for the engines to work properly, they require specific fuels. If the type of fuel given is the wrong blend, the engine will not perform to its maximum capacity. If the fuel is of a poor grade, the engine may sputter, hesitate, and lose power. If the engine is given no fuel at all, it will stop.

The fuel we give our bodies' engines comes directly from the things we consume. The foods we eat contain nutrients. These nutrients come in the form of vitamins, minerals, enzymes, water, amino acids, carbohydrates, and lipids. It is these nutrients that sustain life by providing us with the basic materials our bodies need to carry on their daily functions.

Individual nutrients differ in form and function, and in the amount needed by the body; however, they are all vital to our health. The actions that involve nutrients take place on microscopic levels, and the specific processes differ greatly. Nutrients are involved in all body processes, from combating infection to repairing tissue to thinking. Although nutrients have different specific functions, their common function is to keep us going.

Research has shown that each part of the body contains high concentrations of certain nutrients. A deficiency of those nutrients will cause the body part to malfunction and eventually break down—and, like dominos, other body parts will follow. To keep this from happening, we need a proper diet and appropriate nutritional supplements. Brain function, memory, skin elasticity, eyesight, energy, the ratio of lean to fat tissue in the body, and overall health are all indications of how well the body is functioning. With the help of the proper nutrients, exercise, and a balanced diet, we can slow the aging process and greatly improve our chances for a healthier and pain-free—and possibly longer—life.

If we do not give ourselves the proper nutrients, we can impair the body's normal functions and cause ourselves great harm. Even if we show no signs of illness, we may not necessarily be healthy. It simply may be that we are not yet exhibiting any overt symptoms of illness. One problem most of us have is that we do not get the nutrients we need from our diets because most of the foods we consume are cooked and/or processed. Cooking at high temperatures and processing destroy vital nutrients the body needs to function properly. The organic raw foods that supply these elements are largely missing from today's diet.

The past decade has brought to light much new knowledge about nutrition and its effects on the body, and the role it plays in disease. Phytochemicals, also known as phytonutrients, are one example of the results of this research. These are compounds present in plants that make the plants biologically active. They are not nutrients in the classic sense, but they are what determines a plant's color, flavor, and ability to resist disease. Researchers have identified literally thousands of phytochemicals and also have developed the technology to extract these chemical compounds and concentrate them into pills, powders, and capsules. These are called nutraceuticals—the newest type of dietary supplement.

Your body's nutritional needs are as unique to you as your appearance is. The first essential step toward wellness, therefore, is to be sure you are getting the correct amounts of the proper nutrients. By understanding the principles of holistic nutrition and knowing what nutrients you need, you can improve the state of your health, ward off disease, and maintain a harmonious balance in the way nature intended. Part One should provide you with a clear understanding of the vitamins, minerals, amino acids, enzymes, phytochemicals, and other nutrients you need, as well as important information on natural food supplements, herbs, and products that enhance nutrient activity. Eating a healthful diet and supplementing your diet with appropriate nutrients will help to assure that your organs, cells, and tissues get the fuel they need to operate properly. The nutrients suggested in this book promote healing and wellness by allowing the body to heal and reinvigorate itself.

xv

Nutrition, Diet, and Wellness

UNDERSTANDING THE BASICS OF NUTRITION

Good nutrition is the foundation of good health. Everyone needs the four basic nutrients—water, carbohydrates, proteins, and fats—as well as vitamins, minerals, and other micronutrients. To be able to choose the proper foods, and to better understand why those foods should be supported with supplements, you need to have a clear idea of the components of a healthy diet.

The Four Basic Nutrients

Water, carbohydrates, proteins, and fats are the basic building blocks of a good diet. By choosing the healthiest forms of each of these nutrients and eating them in the proper balance, you enable your body to function at its optimal level.

WATER The human body is two-thirds water. Water is an essential nutrient that is involved in every function of the body. It helps transport nutrients and waste products in and out of cells. It is necessary for all digestive, absorptive, circulatory, and excretory functions, as well as for the utilization of the water-soluble vitamins. It is also needed for the maintenance of proper body temperature. By drinking an adequate amount of water each day—at least eight 8-ounce glasses—you can ensure that your body has all it needs to maintain good health. (For details on choosing the best water, *see* chapter four—WATER.)

CARBOHYDRATES Carbohydrates supply the body with the energy it needs to function. They are found almost exclusively in plant foods, such as fruits, vegetables, peas, and beans. Milk and milk products are the only foods derived from animals that contain a significant amount of carbohydrates.

Carbohydrates are divided into two groups—simple carbohydrates and complex carbohydrates. *Simple carbohydrates,* sometimes called simple sugars, include fructose (fruit sugar), sucrose (table sugar), and lactose (milk sugar), as well as several other sugars. Fruits are one of the richest natural sources of simple carbohydrates. *Complex carbohydrates* are also made up of sugars, but the sugar molecules are strung together to form longer, more complex chains. Complex carbohydrates include fiber and starches. Foods rich in complex carbohydrates include vegetables, whole grains, peas, and beans.

Carbohydrates are the main source of blood glucose, which is a major fuel for all of the body's cells and the only source of energy for the brain and red blood cells. Except for fiber, which cannot be digested, both simple and complex carbohydrates are converted into glucose. The glucose is then either used directly to provide energy for the body or stored in the liver for future use. If a person consumes more calories than his or her body is using, a portion of the carbohydrates consumed may be stored in the body as fat. Due to complex chemical reactions in the brain, eating carbohydrates has a mild tranquilizing effect, and can be beneficial for people who suffer from seasonal affective disorder and/or depression.

When choosing carbohydrate-rich foods for your diet, always select unrefined foods such as fruits, vegetables, peas, beans, and whole-grain products, as opposed to refined, processed foods such as soft drinks, desserts, candy, and sugar. Refined foods offer few, if any, of the vitamins and minerals that are important to your health. In addition, if eaten in excess, especially over a period of many years, the large amounts of simple carbohydrates found in refined foods can lead to a number of disorders, including diabetes and hypoglycemia (low blood sugar). Yet another problem is that foods high in refined simple sugars often are also high in fats, which should be limited in a healthy diet. This is why such foods—which include most cookies and cakes, as well as many snack foods—are usually loaded with calories.

A word is in order here regarding fiber, a very important form of carbohydrate. Referred to in the past as "roughage," dietary fiber is the part of a plant that is resistant to the body's digestive enzymes. As a result, only a relatively small amount of fiber is digested or metabolized in the stomach or intestines. Instead, most of it moves through the gastrointestinal tract and ends up in the stool.

Although most fiber is not digested, it delivers several important health benefits. First, fiber retains water, resulting in softer and bulkier stools that prevent constipation and hemorrhoids. A high-fiber diet also reduces the risk of colon cancer, perhaps by speeding the rate at which stool passes through the intestine and by keeping the digestive tract clean. In addition, fiber binds with certain substances that would normally result in the production of cholesterol, and eliminates these substances from the body. In this way, a high-fiber diet helps lower blood cholesterol levels, reducing the risk of heart disease.

It is recommended that about 60 percent of your total daily calories come from carbohydrates. If much of your diet consists of healthy complex carbohydrates, you should easily fulfill the recommended daily minimum of 25 grams of fiber.

PROTEIN Protein is essential for growth and development. It provides the body with energy, and is needed for the manufacture of hormones, antibodies, enzymes, and tissues. It also helps maintain the proper acid-alkali balance in the body.

When protein is consumed, the body breaks it down into amino acids, the building blocks of all proteins. Some of the amino acids are designated *nonessential*. This does not mean that they are unnecessary, but rather that they do not have to come from the diet because they can be synthesized by the body from other amino acids. Other amino acids are considered *essential,* meaning that the body cannot synthesize them, and therefore must obtain them from the diet.

Whenever the body *makes* a protein—when it builds muscle, for instance—it needs a variety of amino acids for the protein-making process. These amino acids may come from dietary protein or from the body's own pool of amino acids. If a shortage of amino acids becomes chronic, which can occur if the diet is deficient in essential amino acids, the building of protein in the body stops, and the body suffers. (For more information about amino acids, *see* chapter five—AMINO ACIDS.)

Because of the importance of consuming proteins that provide all of the necessary amino acids, dietary proteins are considered to belong to two different groups, depending on the amino acids they provide. *Complete proteins,* which constitute the first group, contain ample amounts of all of the essential amino acids. These proteins are found in meat, fish, poultry, cheese, eggs, and milk. *Incomplete proteins,* which constitute the second group, contain only some of the essential amino acids. These proteins are found in a variety of foods, including grains, legumes, and leafy green vegetables.

Although it is important to consume the full range of amino acids, both essential and nonessential, it is not necessary to get them from meat, fish, poultry, and other complete-protein foods. In fact, because of their high fat content—as well as the use of antibiotics and other chemicals in the raising of poultry and cattle—most of those foods should be eaten in moderation only. Fortunately, the dietary strategy called *mutual supplementation* enables you to combine partial-protein foods to make *complementary protein*—proteins that supply adequate amounts of all the essential amino acids. For instance, although beans and brown rice are both quite rich in protein, each lacks one or more of the necessary amino acids. However, when you combine beans and brown rice with each other, or when you combine either one with any of a number of protein-rich foods, you form a complete protein that is a high-quality substitute for meat. To make a complete protein, combine *beans* with any one of the following:

- Brown rice
- Corn

- Seeds
- Wheat

- Nuts

Or combine *brown rice* with any one of the following:

- Beans
- Nuts

- Seeds
- Wheat

Most Americans eat too much protein, largely as the result of a diet high in meat and dairy products. However, if you have reduced the amount of meat and dairy foods in your diet, you should make sure to get about 50 grams of protein a day. To make sure that you are getting a great enough variety of amino acids in your diet, add protein-rich foods to meals and snacks as often as possible. Eat bread with nut butters, for instance, or add nuts and seeds to salads and vegetable casseroles. Be aware that a combination of any grains, any nuts and seeds, any legumes (such as beans, peanuts, and peas), and a variety of mixed vegetables will make a complete protein. In addition, cornmeal fortified with the amino acid L-lysine makes a complete protein.

All soybean products, such as tofu and soymilk, are complete proteins. They contain the essential amino acids plus several other nutrients. Available in health food stores, tofu, soy oil, soy flour, soy-based meat substitutes, soy cheese, and many other soy products are healthful ways to complement the meatless diet.

Yogurt is the only animal-derived complete-protein source recommended for frequent use in the diet. Made from milk that is curdled by bacteria, yogurt contains *Lactobacillus acidophilus* and other "friendly" bacteria needed for the digestion of foods and the prevention of many disorders, including candidiasis. Yogurt also contains vitamins A and D, and many of the B-complex vitamins.

Do not buy the sweetened, flavored yogurts that are sold in supermarkets. These products contain added sugar and, often, preservatives. Instead, either purchase fresh unsweetened yogurt from a health food store or make the yogurt yourself, and sweeten it with fruit juices and other wholesome ingredients. Yogurt mak-

5

ers are relatively inexpensive and easy to use, and are available at most health food stores.

FATS Although much attention has been focused on the need to reduce dietary fat, the body does need fat. During infancy and childhood, fat is necessary for normal brain development. Throughout life, it is essential to provide energy and support growth. Fat is, in fact, the most concentrated source of energy available to the body. However, after about two years of age, the body requires only small amounts of fat—much less than is provided by the average American diet. Excessive fat intake is a major causative factor in obesity, high blood pressure, coronary heart disease, and colon cancer, and has been linked to a number of other disorders as well. To understand how fat intake is related to these health problems, it is necessary to understand the different types of fats available and the ways in which these fats act within the body.

Fats are composed of building blocks called fatty acids. There are three major categories of fatty acids—saturated, polyunsaturated, and monounsaturated. These classifications are based on the number of hydrogen atoms in the chemical structure of a given molecule of fatty acid.

Saturated fatty acids are found primarily in animal products, including dairy items, such as whole milk, cream, and cheese, and fatty meats like beef, veal, lamb, pork, and ham. The fat marbling you can see in beef and pork is composed of saturated fat. Some vegetable products—including coconut oil, palm kernel oil, and vegetable shortening—are also high in saturates.

The liver uses saturated fats to manufacture cholesterol. Therefore, excessive dietary intake of saturated fats can significantly raise the blood cholesterol level, especially the level of low-density lipoproteins (LDLs), or "bad cholesterol." Guidelines issued by the National Cholesterol Education Program (NCEP), and widely supported by most experts, recommend that the daily intake of saturated fats be kept below 10 percent of total caloric intake. However, for people who have severe problems with high blood cholesterol, even that level may be too high.

Polyunsaturated fatty acids are found in greatest abundance in corn, soybean, safflower, and sunflower oils. Certain fish oils are also high in polyunsaturates. Unlike the saturated fats, polyunsaturates may actually lower your total blood cholesterol level. In doing so, however, large amounts of polyunsaturates also have a tendency to reduce your high-density lipoproteins (HDLs)—your "good cholesterol." For this reason—and because, like all fats, polyunsaturates are high in calories for their weight and volume— the NCEP guidelines state that an individual's intake of polyunsaturated fats should not exceed 10 percent of total caloric intake.

Monounsaturated fatty acids are found mostly in vegetable and nut oils such as olive, peanut, and canola. These fats appear to reduce blood levels of LDLs without affecting HDLs in any way. However, this positive impact upon LDL cholesterol is relatively modest. The NCEP guidelines recommend that intake of monounsaturated fats be kept between 10 and 15 percent of total caloric intake.

Although most foods—including some plant-derived foods— contain a combination of all three types of fatty acids, one of the types usually predominates. Thus, a fat or oil is considered "saturated" or "high in saturates" when it is composed primarily of saturated fatty acids. Such saturated fats are usually solid at room temperature. Similarly, a fat or oil composed mostly of polyunsaturated fatty acids is called "polyunsaturated," while a fat or oil composed mostly of monounsaturated fatty acids is called "monounsaturated."

One other element, *trans-fatty acids,* may play a role in blood cholesterol levels. Also called trans fats, these substances occur when polyunsaturated oils are altered through hydrogenation, a process used to harden liquid vegetable oils into solid foods like margarine and shortening. One recent study found that trans-monounsaturated fatty acids raised LDL cholesterol levels, behaving much like saturated fats. Simultaneously, the trans-fatty acids reduced HDL cholesterol readings. Much more research on this subject is necessary, as studies have not reached consistent and conclusive findings. For now, however, it is clear that if your goal is to lower cholesterol, polyunsaturated and monounsaturted fats are more desirable than saturated fats or products with trans-fatty acids. Just as important, your total calories from fat should not constitute more than 20 to 25 percent of daily calories.

The Micronutrients: Vitamins and Minerals

Like water, carbohydrates, protein, and fats, and the enzymes required to digest them, vitamins and minerals are essential to life. They are therefore considered nutrients, and are often referred to as *micronutrients* simply because they are needed in relatively small amounts compared with the four basic nutrients.

Because vitamins and minerals are so necessary for health, the U.S. Food and Drug Administration (FDA) has formulated recommended consumption levels for vitamins called recommended daily allowances (RDAs). But, as we will see in chapter two—VIT-AMINS—these allowances do not account for the amount needed to maintain maximum health rather than borderline health, only the amount needed to prevent deficiency diseases. Therefore, the average adult who is not suffering from any specific disorder should obtain more than the RDAs of vitamins and minerals from food sources and/or from supplements. The table on page 6—which includes not just vitamin and mineral supplements, but other supplements as well—should be used as a guideline. Although the amounts listed are safe (they will not cause toxicity), they should be varied according to size and weight. People who are active and exercise; those who are under great stress, on restricted diets, or mentally or physically ill; women who take oral contraceptives; those on medication; those who are recovering from surgery; and smokers and those who consume alcoholic beverages all need higher than normal amounts of nutrients.

In addition to a proper diet, exercise and a positive attitude are two important elements that are needed to prevent sickness and disease. If your lifestyle includes each of these, you will feel good and have more energy—something we all deserve. Nature has the answers we need to maintain our health, but you need to know what nutrients you are taking to make sure all the pieces of the puzzle fit together.

NUTRIENTS AND DOSAGES FOR MAINTAINING GOOD HEALTH The nutrients listed below are recommended for good health. Daily dosages are suggested; however, before using any supplements, you should consult with your health care provider. The dosages given here are for adults and children weighing 100 pounds and over. Appropriate dosages for children vary according to age and weight. A child weighing between 70 and 100 pounds should be given three-fourths the adult dose; a child weighing under 70 pounds (and *over* the age of six years) should be given half the adult dose. A child under the age of six years should be given nutritional formulas designed specifically for young children. Follow the dosage directions on the product label.

Use only quality natural (not synthetic) supplements from a reputable source. Lower priced supplements can mean lower quality, with higher levels of fillers and other undesirable ingredients. Give your body the best—it deserves it.

Vitamins	Daily Dosages*
Vitamin A (retinol)	5,000–10,000 IU
A carotenoid complex containing	
beta-carotene	5,000–25,000 IU
Vitamin B_1 (thiamine)	50–100 mg
Vitamin B_2 (riboflavin)	15–50 mg
Vitamin B_3 (niacin)	15–50 mg
(niacinamide)	50–100 mg
Pantothenic acid (vitamin B_5)	50–100 mg
Vitamin B_6 (pyridoxine)	50–100 mg
Vitamin B_{12}	200–400 mcg
Biotin	400–800 mcg
Choline	50–200 mg
Folic acid	400–800 mcg
Inositol	50–200 mg
Para-aminobenzoic acid (PABA)	10–50 mg
Vitamin C with mineral ascorbates	
(Ester-C)	1,000–3,000 mg
Bioflavonoids (mixed)	200–500 mg
Hesperidin	50–100 mg
Rutin	25 mg
Vitamin D_3 (cholecalciferol)	400 IU
Vitamin E (d-alpha-tocopherol)	400–600 IU

Vitamin K (use natural sources such as alfalfa, green leafy vegetables)	100–500 mcg
Essential fatty acids (EFAs) (primrose oil, flaxseed oil, salmon oil, and fish oil are good sources)	As directed on label.

Minerals	**Daily Dosages**
Boron (picolinate or citrate)	3–6 mg
Calcium (citrate, ascorbate, or malate)	1,500–2,000 mg
Chromium (GTF, picolinate, or polynicotinate)	150–400 mcg
Copper	2–3 mg
Iodine (kelp is a good source)	100–225 mcg
Iron** (ferrous gluconate, fumarate, citrate, or amino acid chelate; avoid inorganic forms such as ferrous sulfate, which can oxidize vitamin E.)	18–30 mg
Magnesium	750–1,000 mg
Manganese	3–10 mg
Molybdenum (ascorbate, aspartate, or picolinate)	30–100 mcg
Potassium (citrate)	99–500 mg
Selenium	100–200 mcg
Vanadium (vanadyl sulfate)	200 mcg–1 mg
Zinc	30–50 mg

Amino Acids*	**Daily Dosages**
L-Carnitine	500 mg
Acetyl-L-Carnitine	100–500 mg
L-Cysteine	50–100 mg
Acetyl-L-Cysteine	100–500 mg
L-Lysine	50–100 mg
L-Methionine	50–100 mg
Taurine	100–500 mg
L-Tyrosine	500 mg

Optional Supplements****	**Daily Dosages**
Chondroitin sulfate	As directed on label.
Coenzyme Q_{10}	30–100 mg
Cryptoxanthin	110 mcg

Flavonoids (citrus fruits and berries)	As directed on label.
Garlic	As directed on label.
Ginkgo biloba (herb)	As directed on label.
Glucosamine sulfate	As directed on label.
Lecithin	200–500 mg
Lutein/lycopene	As directed on label.
Pectin	50–100 mg
Phosphatidyl choline	As directed on label.
Phosphatidyl serine	As directed on label.
Pycnogenol or grape seed extract (OPCs)	As directed on label.
Quercetin	70–140 mg
RNA-DNA	100 mg
Silicon	As directed on label.
Soy isoflavones (genistein)	As directed on label.
Superoxide dismutase (SOD)	As directed on label.
Zeaxanthin	90 mcg

*Be careful not to confuse milligrams (mg) with micrograms (mcg). A microgram is $\frac{1}{1,000}$ of a milligram.

**Iron should be taken only if a deficiency exists. Always take iron supplements separately, rather than in a multivitamin and mineral formula.

***See AMINO ACIDS for more information. Individual amino acids should not be taken on a regular basis unless used for treatment of a certain disorder.

****See NATURAL FOOD SUPPLEMENTS for more information.

Other supplements that you may wish to take for increased energy are:

- Bee pollen.
- Coenzyme A.
- Coenzyme 1 (nicotinamide adenine dinucleotide with high-energy hydrogen, or NADH; sold under the brand name Enada).
- Free-form amino acid complex.
- Kyo-Green from Wakunaga of America.
- N,N-Dimethylglycine (DMG).

- Octacosanol.
- Siberian ginseng.
- Spirulina.
- Wheat germ.

In addition, there are many good formulas on the market specifically formulated to help meet the nutritional needs of infants and children, among them Mycel Baby Vites from Ethical Nutrients, a highly absorbable liquid multivitamin formula.

SYNERGY AND DEFICIENCY Data compiled by the U.S. Department of Agriculture indicate that at least 40 percent of the people in this country routinely consume a diet containing only 60 percent of the RDA of each of ten selected nutrients. This means that close to half of the population (and very likely more) suffer from a deficiency of at least one important nutrient. A poll of 37,000 Americans conducted by Food Technology found that half of them were deficient in vitamin B_6 (pyridoxine), 42 percent did not consume sufficient amounts of calcium, 39 percent had an insufficient iron intake, and 25 to 39 percent did not obtain enough vitamin C. Additional research has shown that a vitamin deficiency may not affect the whole body, but only specific cells. For example, those who smoke may suffer from a vitamin C deficiency, but only in the lung area.

Whenever you seek to correct a vitamin or mineral deficiency, you must recognize that nutrients work synergistically. This means that there is a cooperative action between certain vitamins and minerals, which work as catalysts, promoting the absorption and assimilation of other vitamins and minerals. Correcting a deficiency in one vitamin or mineral requires the addition of others, not simply replacement of the one in which you are deficient. This is why taking a single vitamin or mineral may be ineffective, or even dangerous, and why a balanced vitamin and mineral preparation should always be taken in addition to any single supplements. The following table indicates which vitamins and minerals are necessary to correct certain deficiencies.

Vitamin	Supplements Needed for Assimilation
Vitamin A	Choline, essential fatty acids, zinc, vitamins C, D, and E.
Vitamin B complex	Calcium, vitamins C and E.
Vitamin B$_1$ (thiamine)	Manganese, vitamin B complex, vitamins C and E.
Vitamin B$_2$ (riboflavin)	Vitamin B complex, vitamin C.
Vitamin B$_3$ (niacin)	Vitamin B complex, vitamin C.
Pantothenic acid (vitamin B$_5$)	Vitamin B complex, vitamins A, C, and E.
Vitamin B$_6$ (pyridoxine)	Potassium, vitamin B complex, vitamin C.
Biotin	Folic acid, vitamin B complex, pantothenic acid (vitamin B$_5$), vitamin B$_{12}$, vitamin C.
Choline	Vitamin B complex, vitamin B$_{12}$, folic acid, inositol.
Inositol	Vitamin B complex, vitamin C.
Para-aminobenzoic acid (PABA)	Vitamin B complex, folic acid, vitamin C.
Vitamin C	Bioflavonoids, calcium, magnesium.
Vitamin D	Calcium, choline, essential fatty acids, phosphorus, vitamins A and C.
Vitamin E	Essential fatty acids, manganese, selenium, vitamin A, vitamin B$_1$ (thiamine), inositol, vitamin C.
Essential fatty acids	Vitamins A, C, D, and E.

Mineral	Supplements Needed for Assimilation
Calcium	Boron, essential fatty acids, lysine, magnesium, manganese, phosphorus, vitamins A, C, D, and E.
Copper	Cobalt, folic acid, iron, zinc.
Iodine	Iron, manganese, phosphorus.
Magnesium	Calcium, phosphorus, potassium, vitamin B$_6$ (pyridoxine), vitamins C and D.

Manganese	Calcium, iron, vitamin B complex, vitamin E.
Phosphorus	Calcium, iron, manganese, sodium, vitamin B_6 (pyridoxine).
Silicon	Iron, phosphorus.
Sodium	Calcium, potassium, sulfur, vitamin D.
Sulfur	Potassium, vitamin B_1 (thiamine), pantothenic acid (vitamin B_5), biotin.
Zinc	Calcium, copper, phosphorus, vitamin B_6 (pyridoxine).

There are certain cautions that you should take into account when taking supplements. Antibiotics interfere with the natural balance of normal intestinal flora needed to produce vitamin K, which is necessary for normal blood clotting and maintaining the integrity of the bones. Too much coffee and/or caffeinated soft drinks can interfere with calcium metabolism. Aspirin can irritate the gastrointestinal tract, and may cause gastrointestinal bleeding. Aspirin can also interfere with the absorption of B vitamins and vitamin C. If you are taking aspirin daily for cardiovascular health, it is better to take baby aspirin—studies have shown that it is less irritating to the gastrointestinal tract, and it works just as well as ordinary aspirin.

GUIDELINES FOR SELECTING AND PREPARING FOODS

Clearly, a healthy diet must provide a proper balance of the four essential nutrients, as well as a rich supply of vitamins, minerals, and other micronutrients. However, it is not enough simply to purchase foods that are high in complex carbohydrates, fiber, and complementary proteins, and low in saturated fats. Food also must be free of harmful additives, and it must be prepared in a way that preserves its nutrients and avoids the production of harmful substances.

When nutritionists talk about diet, they are referring to live whole foods—unprocessed food with nothing added or taken away. Whole foods are more healthful because they contain no potentially harmful ingredients. In addition, plant foods are full of hundreds of phytochemicals that can help prevent disease and keep the body healthy. These are our front-line defenders against cancer and free radicals (*see* Phytochemicals, page 18). Foods known to supply important phytochemicals include soybeans and soy products, broccoli, citrus peels, flax, garlic, green tea, grapes, and tomatoes.

Avoid Foods That Contain Additives and Artificial Ingredients

Additives are placed in foods for a number of reasons: to lengthen shelf life; to make a food more appealing by enhancing color, texture, or taste; to facilitate food preparation; or to otherwise make the product more marketable. Certain additives, like sugar, are derived from natural sources. Other additives, like aspartame (NutraSweet), are made synthetically.

Although many additives are used in very small amounts, it has been estimated that the average American consumes about 5 pounds of additives per year. If you include sugar—the food-processing industry's most used additive—the number jumps to 135 pounds a year. Anyone whose diet is high in processed products clearly consumes a significant amount of additives and artificial ingredients.

At their best, additives and artificial ingredients simply add little or no nutritional value to a food product. At their worst, additives pose a threat to your health. The history of additive use includes a number of products that were once deemed safe but later were banned or allowed to be used only if accompanied by warnings. The artificial sweeteners cyclamate and saccharin are just two examples of such products. Other additives, like monosodium glutamate (MSG) and aspartame, are used without warnings, but have been known to cause problems ranging from headaches and diarrhea to confusion, memory loss, and seizures.

The number of food additives now in use is staggering. To learn more about these substances, you can consult Michael Jacobson's *Safe Food: Eating Wisely in a Risky World* (Living Planet Press, 1991) or *Unsafe at Any Meal* by Earl Mindell (Warner Books, 1986).

Increase Your Consumption of Raw Produce

The most healthful fruits and vegetables are those that have been grown organically—without the use of insecticides, herbicides, artificial fertilizers, or growth-stimulating chemicals. Organic produce can be found in select health food stores, as well as in some supermarkets and greenmarkets and through food co-ops.

When choosing your produce, look for fruits and vegetables that are at the peak of ripeness. These contain more vitamins and enzymes than do foods that are underripe or overripe, or that have been stored for any length of time. Remember that the longer a food is kept in storage, the more nutrients it loses.

Once you get your organic produce home, running water and a vegetable brush are probably all that will be needed to get it ready for the table. If the produce is not organic, however, you will want to wash it more thoroughly to rid it of any chemical residues. Use a soft vegetable brush to scrub the foods, and then let them soak in water for ten minutes. You can also clean produce with nontoxic rinsing preparations, which are available in reputable health food stores. If the products are waxed, peel them, as wax cannot be washed away, but remove as thin a layer of peel as possible.

Most fruits and vegetables should be eaten in their entirety, as all of the parts, including the skin, contain valuable nutrients. When eating citrus fruits, remove the rinds, but eat the white part inside the skin for its vitamin C and bioflavonoid content.

Although most people usually cook their vegetables before eating, both fruits and vegetables should be eaten raw as much as possible. All enzymes and most vitamins are extremely sensitive to heat, and are usually destroyed in the cooking process.

If fresh produce is unavailable, use frozen foods instead. Do not use canned vegetables or boxed vegetable dishes, as they usually contain significant amounts of salt and other unhealthy additives. If raw produce does not agree with you, steam your vegetables lightly in a steamer, cooking pan, or wok just until slightly tender.

Avoid Overcooking Your Foods

As just discussed, cooking foods for all but brief periods of time can destroy many valuable nutrients. More alarming is that when foods are cooked to the point of browning or charring, the organic compounds they contain undergo changes in structure, producing carcinogens.

Barbecued meats seem to pose the worst health threat in this regard. When burning fat drips onto an open flame, polycyclic aromatic hydrocarbons (PAHs)—dangerous carcinogens—are formed. When amino acids and other chemicals found in muscle are exposed to high temperatures, other carcinogens, called heterocyclic aromatic amines (HAAs), are created. In fact, many of the chemicals used to produce cancer in laboratory animals have been isolated from cooked proteins.

It is important to note, though, that cooked meats do not pose the only threat. Even browned or burned bread crusts contain a variety of carcinogenic substances.

The dangers posed by the practice of cooking foods at high temperatures or until browned or burned should not be dismissed. Although eating habits vary widely from person to person, it seems safe to assume that many people consume many grams of overcooked foods a day. By comparison, only half a gram of this same dangerous burned material is inhaled by someone who smokes two packs of cigarettes a day. Clearly, by eating produce raw or only lightly cooked, and by greatly limiting your consumption of meat, you will be doing much to decrease your risk of cancer and, possibly, other disorders.

Use the Proper Cooking Utensils

Although raw foods have many advantages over cooked, nourishing soups and a variety of other dishes can be made healthfully. One of the ways to ensure wholesome cooked food is the careful selection of cookware.

When preparing foods, use only glass, stainless steel, or iron pots and pans. Do not use aluminum cookware or utensils. Foods cooked or stored in aluminum produce a substance that neutral-

PHYTOCHEMICALS

For many years, researchers have recognized that diets high in fruits, vegetables, grains, and legumes appear to reduce the risk of a number of diseases, including cancer, heart disease, diabetes, and high blood pressure when compared with diets high in meat. More recently, it was discovered that the disease-preventing effects of these foods are partly due to antioxidants—specific vitamins, minerals, and enzymes that help prevent cancer and other disorders by protecting cells against damage from oxidation. Now, researchers have discovered that fruits, vegetables, grains, and legumes contain yet another group of health-promoting nutrients. Called *phytochemicals,* these substances appear to be powerful ammunition in the war against cancer and other disorders.

Phytochemicals are the biologically active substances in plants that are responsible for giving them color, flavor, and natural disease resistance. To understand how phytochemicals protect the body against cancer, it is necessary to understand that cancer formation is a multistep process. Phytochemicals seem to fight cancer by blocking one or more of the steps that lead to cancer. For instance, cancer can begin when a carcinogenic molecule—from the food you eat or the air you breathe—invades a cell. But if sulforaphane, a phytochemical found in broccoli, also reaches the cell, it activates a group of enzymes that whisk the carcinogen out of the cell before it can cause any harm.

Other phytochemicals are known to prevent cancer in other ways. Flavonoids, found in citrus fruits and berries, keep cancer-causing hormones from latching on to cells in the first place. Genistein, found in soybeans, kills tumors by preventing the formation of the capillaries needed to nourish them. Indoles, found in cruciferous vegetables such as Brussels sprouts, cauliflower, and cabbage, increase immune activity and make it easier for the body to excrete toxins. Saponins, found in kidney beans, chickpeas, soybeans, and lentils, may prevent cancer cells from multiplying. P-coumaric acid and chlorogenic acid, found in tomatoes, interfere with certain chemical unions that can create

izes the digestive juices, leading to acidosis and ulcers. Worse, the aluminum in the cookware can leach from the pot into the food. When the food is consumed, the aluminum is absorbed by the carcinogens. The list of these protective substances goes on and on. Tomatoes alone are believed to contain an estimated 10,000 different phytochemicals.

Although no long-term human studies have shown that specific phytochemicals stop cancer, research on phytochemicals supports the more than 200 studies that link lowered cancer risk with a diet rich in grains, legumes, fruits, and vegetables. Moreover, animal and in vitro studies have demonstrated how some phytochemicals prevent carcinogens from promoting the growth of specific cancers. For instance, the phytochemical phenethyl isothiocyanate (PEITC), found in cabbage and turnips, has been shown to inhibit the growth of lung cancer in rats and mice. Among other things, PEITC protects the cells' DNA from a potent carcinogen found in tobacco smoke.

Researchers have been able to isolate some phytochemicals, and a number of companies are now selling concentrates that contain phytochemicals obtained from vegetables such as broccoli. These may be used as supplemental sources of some of these nutrients. However, such pills should *not* be seen as replacements for fresh whole foods. Because several *thousand* phytochemicals are currently known to exist, and because new ones are being discovered all the time, no supplement can possibly contain all of the cancer-fighters found in a shopping basket full of fruits and vegetables.

Fortunately, it is easy to get a healthy dose of phytochemicals at every meal. Almost every grain, legume, fruit, and vegetable tested has been found to contain these substances. Moreover, unlike many vitamins, these substances do not appear to be destroyed by cooking or other processing. Genistein, the substance found in soybeans, for instance, is also found in soybean products such as tofu and miso soup. Similarly, the phytochemical PEITC, found in cabbage, remains intact even when the cabbage is made into cole slaw or sauerkraut. Of course, by eating much of your produce raw or only lightly cooked, you will be able to enjoy the benefits not just of phytochemicals, but of all of the vitamins, minerals, and other nutrients that fresh whole foods have to offer.

19

body, where it accumulates in the brain and nervous system tissues. Excessive amounts of these aluminum deposits have been implicated in Alzheimer's disease.

BASIC NUTRITIONAL GUIDE

A diet high in nutrients is the key to good health. Use the following section as a guide when deciding which types of food to include in your diet and which ones to avoid in order to maintain good health.

Beans

FOODS TO AVOID Canned pork and beans, canned beans with salt or preservatives, frozen beans.

ACCEPTABLE FOODS All beans (especially soy) cooked without animal fat or salt.

Beverages

FOODS TO AVOID Alcoholic drinks, coffee, cocoa, pasteurized and/or sweetened juices and fruit drinks, sodas, tea (except herbal tea).

ACCEPTABLE FOODS Herbal teas, fresh vegetable and fruit juices, cereal grain beverages (often sold as coffee substitutes), mineral or distilled water.

Dairy products

FOODS TO AVOID All soft cheeses, all pasteurized or artificially colored cheese products, ice cream.

ACCEPTABLE FOODS Raw goat cheese, nonfat cottage cheese, kefir, unsweetened yogurt, goat's milk, raw or skim milk, buttermilk.

Eggs

FOODS TO AVOID Fried or pickled.

ACCEPTABLE FOODS Boiled or poached (limit of four weekly).

Fish

FOODS TO AVOID All fried fish, all shellfish, salted fish, anchovies, herring, fish canned in oil.

ACCEPTABLE FOODS All freshwater white fish, salmon, broiled or baked fish, water-packed tuna.

Other cookware to be avoided includes all pots and pans with nonstick coatings. Too often, the metals and other substances in the pots' finish flakes or leaches into the food. Ultimately, these chemicals end up in your body.

Fruits

FOODS TO AVOID Canned, bottled, or frozen fruits with sweeteners added; oranges.

ACCEPTABLE FOODS All fresh, frozen, stewed, or dried fruits without sweeteners (except oranges, which are acidic and highly allergenic), unsulfured fruits, home-canned fruits.

Grains

FOODS TO AVOID All white flour products, white rice, pasta, crackers, cold cereals, instant types of oatmeal and other hot cereals.

ACCEPTABLE FOODS All whole grains and products containing whole grains: cereals, breads, muffins, whole-grain crackers, cream of wheat or rye cereal, buckwheat, millet, oats, brown rice, wild rice. (Limit yeast breads to three servings per week.)

Meats

FOODS TO AVOID Beef; all forms of pork; hot dogs; luncheon meats; smoked, pickled, and processed meats; corned beef; duck; goose; spare ribs; gravies; organ meats.

ACCEPTABLE FOODS Skinless turkey and chicken, lamb. (Limit meat to three 3-oz servings per week.)

Nuts

FOODS TO AVOID All salted or roasted nuts; peanuts (if suffering from any disorder).

ACCEPTABLE FOODS All fresh raw nuts (peanuts in moderation only).

Oils (fats)

FOODS TO AVOID All saturated fats, hydrogenated margarine, refined processed oils, shortenings, hardened oils.

ACCEPTABLE FOODS All cold-pressed oils: corn, safflower, sesame, olive, flaxseed, soybean, sunflower, and canola oils; margarine made from these oils; eggless mayonnaise.

continued on next page.

21

Limit Your Use of Salt

Although some sodium is essential for survival, inadequate sodium intake is a rare problem. We need less than 500 milligrams of sodium a day to stay healthy. This is enough to accomplish all the vital functions that sodium performs in the body—helping main-

continued from previous page

Seasonings

FOODS TO AVOID Black or white pepper, salt, hot red peppers, all types of vinegar except pure natural apple cider vinegar.

ACCEPTABLE FOODS Garlic, onions, cayenne, Spike, all herbs, dried vegetables, apple cider vinegar, tamari, miso, seaweed, dulse.

Soups

FOODS TO AVOID Canned soups made with salt, preservatives, MSG, or fat stock; all creamed soups.

ACCEPTABLE FOODS Homemade (salt- and fat-free) bean, lentil, pea, vegetable, barley, brown rice, onion.

Sprouts and seeds

FOODS TO AVOID All seeds cooked in oil or salt.

ACCEPTABLE FOODS All slightly cooked sprouts (except alfalfa, which should be raw and washed thoroughly), wheatgrass, all raw seeds.

Sweets

FOODS TO AVOID White, brown, or raw cane sugar, corn syrups, chocolate, sugar candy, fructose (except that in fresh whole fruit), all syrups (except pure maple syrup), all sugar substitutes, jams and jellies made with sugar.

ACCEPTABLE FOODS Barley malt or rice syrup, small amounts of raw honey, pure maple syrup, stevia, unsulfured blackstrap molasses.

Vegetables

FOODS TO AVOID All canned or frozen with salt or additives.

ACCEPTABLE FOODS All raw, fresh, frozen (no additives), or home-canned without salt (undercook vegetables slightly).

tain normal fluid levels, healthy muscle function, and proper acidity (pH) of the blood. Excessive sodium intake can cause fluid to be retained in the tissues, which can lead to hypertension (high blood pressure) and can aggravate many medical disorders, including congestive heart failure, certain forms of kidney disease, and premenstrual syndrome (PMS).

One of the best ways to limit the sodium in your diet is to limit your use of salt when cooking and dining. Just as important, stay away from processed foods, which often contain excessively high amounts of sodium.

Vitamins

INTRODUCTION

Vitamins are essential to life. They contribute to good health by regulating the metabolism and assisting the biochemical processes that release energy from digested food. They are considered micronutrients because the body needs them in relatively small amounts compared with nutrients such as carbohydrates, proteins, fats, and water.

Enzymes are essential chemicals that are the foundation of human bodily functions. (*See* chapter seven—ENZYMES.) They are catalysts (activators) in the chemical reactions that are continually taking place within the body. As coenzymes, vitamins work with enzymes, thereby allowing all the activities that occur within the body to be carried out as they should. Whole, fresh raw foods are a good source of enzymes.

Of the major vitamins, some are water soluble and some are oil soluble. Water-soluble vitamins must be taken into the body daily, as they cannot be stored and are excreted within four hours to one day. These include vitamin C and the B-complex vitamins. Oil-soluble vitamins can be stored for longer periods of time in the body's fatty tissue and the liver. These include vitamins A, D, E, and K. Both types of vitamins are needed by the body for proper functioning.

RDA VERSUS RDI VERSUS ODI

Recommended Dietary Allowances (RDAs) were instituted over forty years ago by the National Academy of Sciences' U.S. Food and Nutrition Board as a standard for the daily amounts of vitamins needed by a healthy person. These RDAs were the basis for the U.S. Recommended Daily Allowances (U.S. RDAs) adopted by the Food and Drug Administration (FDA). The provisions of the Nutrition Labeling and Education Act and the Dietary Supplement Act of 1992 required a change in food product labeling to use a new reference term, Daily Value (DV), which began to appear on FDA-regulated product labels in 1994.

DVs are made up of two sets of references: Daily Reference Values (DRVs) and Reference Daily Intakes (RDIs). DRVs are a set of dietary references that apply to fat, saturated fat, cholesterol, carbohydrate, protein, fiber, sodium, and potassium. RDIs are a set of dietary references based on the Recommended Dietary Allowances for essential vitamins and minerals and, in selected groups, protein. The term *RDI* replaces *U.S. RDA*.

Unfortunately, the amounts of these nutrients defined by the Recommended Dietary Allowances give us only the bare minimum required to ward off vitamin deficiency diseases such as beriberi, rickets, scurvy, and night blindness. What they do not account for are the amounts needed to maintain maximum health, rather than borderline health.

Scientific studies have shown that taking dosages of vitamins above the RDIs helps our bodies work better. The RDIs therefore are not very useful for determining what our intake of different vitamins should be. We prefer to speak in terms of *optimum daily intakes* (ODIs)—the amounts of nutrients needed for vibrant good health. This entails consuming larger amounts of vitamins than the RDIs. The nutrient doses recommended on page 9 are ODIs. By providing our bodies with an optimum daily amount of necessary vitamins, we can enhance our health. The dosages outlined in this book will enable you to design a vitamin program that is custom-tailored for the individual.

25

BALANCE AND SYNERGY

Having the proper balance of vitamins and minerals is very important. Scientific research has proved that excesses of isolated vitamins or minerals can produce the same symptoms as deficiencies of vitamins or minerals. For example, high doses of isolated B vitamins have been shown to cause the depletion of other B vitamins. Similarly, if zinc is taken in excess, symptoms of zinc deficiency can result. Studies have shown that an intake of up to 100 milligrams of zinc daily enhances immune function, but an amount in excess of 100 milligrams daily may actually harm immune function.

Synergy is a phenomenon whereby two or more vitamins combine to create a stronger vitamin function than the sum of their individual effects would suggest. For example, in order for bioflavonoids to work properly (they prevent bruising and bleeding gums), they must be taken along with vitamin C. Recent studies show that bioflavonoids also may be a big factor in preventing cancer and many other diseases.

In addition, certain substances can block the absorption and effects of vitamins. For example, the absorption of vitamin C is greatly reduced by antibiotic drugs, so a person taking antibiotics requires a higher than normal intake of this vitamin.

SYNTHETIC VERSUS NATURAL

Ideally, all of us would get all of the nutrients we need for optimal health from fresh, healthful foods. In reality, however, this is often difficult, if not impossible. In our chemically polluted and stress-filled world, our nutritional requirements have been increasing, but the number of calories we require has been *decreasing,* as our general level of physical activity has declined. This means we are faced with needing somehow to get more nutrients from less food. At the same time, many of our foods are depleted of certain nutrients. Modern farming practices have resulted in soils that are lacking in selenium and other nutrients. Harvesting and shipping practices are dictated not by nutritional considerations but by marketing demands. Add to this extensive processing, improper storage, and other factors, and it is little wonder that many of the foods that reach our tables cannot meet our nutritional needs. Getting even the RDIs of vitamins from today's diet has become quite hard to do. This means that for optimum health, it is necessary to take nutrients in supplement form.

Vitamin supplements can be divided into two groups: synthetic and natural. Synthetic vitamins are vitamins produced in laboratories from isolated chemicals that mirror their counterparts found in nature. Natural vitamins are derived from food sources. Although there are no major chemical differences between a vitamin found in food and one created in a laboratory, synthetic supplements contain the isolated vitamins only, while natural supplements may contain other nutrients not yet discovered. This is because these vitamins are in their natural state. If you are deficient in a particular nutrient, the chemical source will work, but you will not get the benefits of the vitamin as found in whole foods. Supplements that are not labeled natural also may include coal tars, artificial coloring, preservatives, sugars, and starch, as well as other additives. You should beware of such harmful elements. However, you should also note that a bottle of "natural" vitamins may contain vitamins that have not been extracted from a natural food source. It is necessary to read labels carefully to make sure the products you buy contain nutrients from food sources, with none of the artificial additives mentioned above.

Studies have shown that protein-bonded vitamins, as found in natural whole food supplements, are absorbed, utilized, and retained in the tissues better than supplements that are not protein-bonded. Chemical-derived vitamins are not protein-bonded. Vitamins and minerals in food are bonded to proteins, lipids, carbohydrates, and bioflavonoids. Dr. Abram Hoffer, one of the "founding fathers" of orthomolecular medicine (a school of medicine that emphasizes the role of nutrition in health), explains:

Components [of food] do not exist free in nature; nature does not lay down pure protein, pure fat, or pure carbohydrates. Their molecules are interlaced in very complex three-dimensional structures which even now have not been fully described. Intermingled are the essential nutrients such as vitamins and minerals, again not free, but combined in complex molecules.

Using a natural form of vitamins and minerals in nutritional supplements is the objective of the protein-bonding process. Taking supplements with meals helps to assure a supply of other nutrients needed for better assimilation as well.

WHAT'S ON THE SHELVES

Over-the-counter vitamin supplements come in various forms, combinations, and amounts. They are available in tablet, capsule, gel-capsule, powder, sublingual, lozenge, and liquid forms. They can also be administered by injection. In most cases, it is a matter of personal preference as to how you take them; however, due to slight variations in how rapidly the supplements are absorbed and assimilated into the body, we will sometimes recommend one form over another. These recommendations are given throughout the book.

Vitamin supplements are usually available as isolated vitamins or in combination with other nutrients. It is important to select your vitamins based upon what you really need. A program designed for health maintenance would be different from one designed to overcome a specific disorder. If you find one supplement that meets your needs, remember to take it daily. If it does not contain a large enough quantity of what you want, you may consider taking more than one. Just make sure that you are aware of the increased dosage of the other nutrients it may contain. If there is no single supplement that provides you with what you are looking for, consider taking a combination of different supplements. This book lists each supplement separately, so you will know what each does and the amount needed. But you may find a supplement that contains several needed nutrients in one tablet or capsule.

Because the potency of most vitamins may be decreased by sunlight, make sure that the container holding your vitamins is dark enough to shield its contents properly. Some people may be sensitive to plastic, and may need to purchase vitamins in glass containers. Vitamin supplements should be kept in a cool, dark place.

All vitamin supplements work best when taken in combination with food. Unless specified otherwise, oil-soluble vitamins should be taken before meals, and water-soluble ones should be taken after meals.

VITAMINS FROM A TO Z

Vitamin A and the Carotenoids

Vitamin A prevents night blindness and other eye problems, as well as some skin disorders, such as acne. It enhances immunity, may help to heal gastrointestinal ulcers, and is needed for the maintenance and repair of epithelial tissue, of which the skin and mucous membranes are composed. It is important in the formation of bones and teeth, aids in fat storage, and protects against colds, flu, and infections of the kidneys, bladder, lungs, and mucous membranes. Vitamin A acts as an antioxidant, helping to protect the cells against cancer and other diseases (*see* chapter six—ANTI-OXIDANTS) and is necessary for new cell growth. It guards against heart disease and stroke, and lowers cholesterol levels. This important vitamin also slows the aging process. Protein cannot be utilized by the body without vitamin A. Vitamin A is a well-known wrinkle eliminator. Applied topically in the form of tretinoin (the active ingredient in Retin-A and Renova), vitamin A reduces fine lines in the skin and helps fade age spots.

A deficiency of vitamin A can cause dry hair and/or skin, dryness of the conjunctiva and cornea, poor growth, and/or night blindness. Other possible results of vitamin A deficiency include abscesses in the ears; insomnia; fatigue; reproductive difficulties; sinusitis, pneumonia, and frequent colds and other respiratory infections; skin disorders, including acne; and weight loss.

The *carotenoids* are a class of compounds related to vitamin A. In some cases, they can act as precursors of vitamin A; some act as antioxidants or have other important functions. The best known

29

subclass of the carotenoids are the carotenes, of which beta-carotene is the most widely known. Also included in this group are alpha- and gamma-carotene, and lycopene. When food or supplements containing beta-carotene are consumed, the beta-carotene is converted into vitamin A in the liver. According to recent reports, beta-carotene appears to aid in cancer prevention by scavenging, or neutralizing, free radicals. Other types of carotenoids that have been identified are the xanthophylls (including beta-cryptoxanthin, canthaxanthin, lutein, and zeaxanthin); the limonoids (including limonene); and the phytosterols (including perillyl alcohol). Science has not yet discovered all of the carotenoids, although one source documents 563 different carotenoids identified so far. Combinations of carotenoids have been shown to be more beneficial than individual carotenoids taken alone.

Taking large amounts of vitamin A, over 100,000 international units daily, over long periods can be toxic to the body, mainly the liver. Toxic levels of vitamin A are associated with abdominal pain, amenorrhea (cessation of menstruation), enlargement of the liver and/or spleen, gastrointestinal disturbances, hair loss, itching, joint pain, nausea and vomiting, water on the brain, elevated liver enzymes, and small cracks and scales on the lips and at the corners of the mouth. Excessive intake of vitamin A during pregnancy has been linked to birth defects, including cleft palate and heart defects. It is better to take beta-carotene during pregnancy. If you have a particular disorder that calls for taking high doses of vitamin A, use an emulsified form, which puts less stress on the liver.

No overdose can occur with beta-carotene, although if you take too much, your skin may turn slightly yellow-orange in color. Beta-carotene does not have the same effect as vitamin A in the body and is not harmful in larger amounts unless your liver cannot convert beta-carotene into vitamin A. People with hypothyroidism often have this problem. It is important to take only *natural* beta-carotene or a natural carotenoid complex. Betatene is the trade name for a type of carotenoid complex extracted from sea algae. It is used as an ingredient in various products by different manufacturers.

SOURCES Vitamin A can be found in animal livers, fish liver oils, and green and yellow fruits and vegetables. Foods that contain significant amounts include apricots, asparagus, beet greens, broccoli, cantaloupe, carrots, collards, dandelion greens, dulse, fish liver and fish liver oil, garlic, kale, mustard greens, papayas, peaches, pumpkin, red peppers, spinach, spirulina, sweet potatoes, Swiss chard, turnip greens, watercress, and yellow squash. It is also present in the following herbs: alfalfa, borage leaves, burdock root, cayenne (capsicum), chickweed, eyebright, fennel seed, hops, horsetail, kelp, lemongrass, mullein, nettle, oat straw, paprika, parsley, peppermint, plantain, raspberry leaf, red clover, rose hips, sage, uva ursi, violet leaves, watercress, and yellow dock. Animal sources of vitamin A are up to six times as strong as vegetable sources.

COMMENTS Antibiotics, laxatives, and some cholesterol-lowering drugs interfere with the absorption of vitamin A.

CAUTIONS If you have liver disease, do not take a daily dose of over 10,000 international units of vitamin A in pill form, or any amount of cod liver oil. If you are pregnant, do not take more than 10,000 international units of vitamin A daily because of reported problems in fetal development. Children should not take more than 18,000 international units of vitamin A on a daily basis for over one month. For most people, beta-carotene is the best source of vitamin A because it is converted by the liver into only the amount of vitamin A that the body actually needs. However, if you have diabetes or hypothyroidism, there is a good possibility your body cannot convert beta-carotene into vitamin A. Consuming large amounts of beta-carotene may therefore place unnecessary stress on your liver.

Vitamin B Complex

The B vitamins help to maintain the health of the nerves, skin, eyes, hair, liver, and mouth, as well as healthy muscle tone in the gastrointestinal tract and proper brain function. B-complex vitamins act as coenzymes, helping enzymes to react chemically with other substances, and are involved in energy production. They may be useful for alleviating depression or anxiety as well. Adequate intake of the B vitamins is very important for elderly people because these nutrients are not as well absorbed as we age. There have even been cases of people diagnosed with Alzheimer's disease whose problems were later found to be due to a deficiency of vitamin B_{12} plus the B complex. The B vitamins should always be taken together, but up to two to three times more of one B vitamin than another can be taken for a period of time if needed for a particular disorder. There are spray and sublingual forms that are absorbed more easily, which are good choices for older adults and those with absorption problems.

Because the B vitamins work together, a deficiency in one often indicates a deficiency in another. Although the B vitamins are a team, they will be discussed individually.

Vitamin B₁ (Thiamine)

Thiamine enhances circulation and assists in blood formation, carbohydrate metabolism, and the production of hydrochloric acid, which is important for proper digestion. Thiamine also optimizes cognitive activity and brain function. It has a positive effect on energy, growth, normal appetite, and learning capacity, and is needed for proper muscle tone of the intestines, stomach, and heart. Thiamine also acts as an antioxidant, protecting the body from the degenerative effects of aging, alcohol consumption, and smoking.

Beriberi, a nervous system disease that is rare in developed nations, is caused by a deficiency of thiamine. Other symptoms that can result from thiamine deficiency include constipation, edema, enlarged liver, fatigue, forgetfulness, gastrointestinal disturbances, heart changes, irritability, labored breathing, loss of appetite, muscle atrophy, nervousness, numbness of the hands and feet, pain and sensitivity, poor coordination, tingling sensations, weak and sore muscles, general weakness, and severe weight loss.

SOURCES The richest food sources of thiamine include brown rice, egg yolks, fish, legumes, liver, peanuts, peas, pork, poultry, rice bran, wheat germ, and whole grains. Other sources are asparagus, brewer's yeast, broccoli, Brussels sprouts, dulse, kelp, most nuts, oatmeal, plums, dried prunes, raisins, spirulina, and watercress. Herbs that contain thiamine include alfalfa, bladderwrack, burdock root, catnip, cayenne, chamomile, chickweed, eyebright, fennel seed, fenugreek, hops, nettle, oat straw, parsley, peppermint, raspberry leaf, red clover, rose hips, sage, yarrow, and yellow dock.

COMMENTS Antibiotics, phenytoin (Dilantin, a drug used to prevent seizures), sulfa drugs, and oral contraceptives, and heavy alcohol or caffeine consumption may decrease thiamine levels in the body. A high-carbohydrate diet increases the need for thiamine. Alcoholics are among those most often deficient in thiamine.

Vitamin B₂ (Riboflavin)

Riboflavin is necessary for red blood cell formation, antibody production, cell respiration, and growth. It alleviates eye fatigue and is important in the prevention and treatment of cataracts. It aids in the metabolism of carbohydrates, fats, and proteins. Together with vitamin A, it maintains and improves the mucous membranes in the digestive tract. Riboflavin also facilitates the use of oxygen by the tissues of the skin, nails, and hair; eliminates dandruff; and helps the absorption of iron and vitamin B₆ (pyridoxine). Consumption of adequate amounts of riboflavin is important during pregnancy, because a lack of this vitamin can damage a developing fetus even if a woman shows no signs of deficiency. Riboflavin is needed for the metabolism of the amino acid tryptophan, which is converted into niacin in the body. Carpal tunnel syndrome may benefit from a treatment program that includes riboflavin and vitamin B₆.

Deficiency symptoms include cracks and sores at the corners of the mouth, eye disorders, inflammation of the mouth and tongue, and skin lesions, a group of symptoms collectively referred to as *ariboflavinosis*. Other possible deficiency symptoms include dermatitis, dizziness, hair loss, insomnia, light sensitivity, poor digestion, retarded growth, and slowed mental response.

SOURCES High levels of vitamin B₂ are found in the following foods: cheese, egg yolks, fish, legumes, meat, milk, poultry, spinach, whole grains, and yogurt. Other sources include aspara-

33

gus, avocados, broccoli, Brussels sprouts, currants, dandelion greens, dulse, kelp, leafy green vegetables, mushrooms, molasses, nuts, and watercress. Herbs that contain vitamin B$_2$ include alfalfa, bladderwrack, burdock root, catnip, cayenne, chamomile, chickweed, eyebright, fennel seed, fenugreek, ginseng, hops, horsetail, mullein, nettle, oat straw, parsley, peppermint, raspberry leaves, red clover, rose hips, sage, and yellow dock.

COMMENTS Factors that increase the need for riboflavin include the use of oral contraceptives and strenuous exercise. This B vitamin is easily destroyed by light, antibiotics, and alcohol. Taking too much riboflavin (over 50 milligrams daily) over a long period of time may lead to cataracts and retinal diseases.

Vitamin B$_3$ (Niacin, Nicotinic Acid, Niacinamide)

Vitamin B$_3$ is needed for proper circulation and healthy skin. It aids in the functioning of the nervous system; in the metabolism of carbohydrates, fats, and proteins; and in the production of hydrochloric acid for the digestive system. It is involved in the normal secretion of bile and stomach fluids, and in the synthesis of sex hormones. Niacin lowers cholesterol and improves circulation. It is helpful for schizophrenia and other mental illnesses, and is also a memory-enhancer.

Pellagra is a disease caused by niacin deficiency. Other symptoms of niacin deficiency include canker sores, dementia, depression, diarrhea, dizziness, fatigue, halitosis, headaches, indigestion, insomnia, limb pains, loss of appetite, low blood sugar, muscular weakness, skin eruptions, and inflammation.

SOURCES Niacin and niacinamide are found in beef liver, brewer's yeast, broccoli, carrots, cheese, corn flour, dandelion greens, dates, eggs, fish, milk, peanuts, pork, potatoes, tomatoes, wheat germ, and whole wheat products. Herbs that contain niacin include alfalfa, burdock root, catnip, cayenne, chamomile, chickweed, eyebright, fennel seed, hops, licorice, mullein, nettle, oat straw, parsley, peppermint, raspberry leaf, red clover, rose hips, slippery elm, and yellow dock.

COMMENTS A flush, usually harmless, may occur after the ingestion of niacin supplements; a red rash appears on the skin and a tingling sensation may be experienced as well. Usually, these symptoms last only a few minutes. There are two forms of this vitamin: niacin (or nicotinic acid) and niacinamide. In the form of niacinamide, it does not cause flushing. However, niacinamide does not have all the same properties of niacin. Specifically, it is not effective for lowering blood cholesterol.

CAUTIONS People who are pregnant or who suffer from diabetes, glaucoma, gout, liver disease, or peptic ulcers should use niacin supplements with caution. Niacin may elevate blood sugar levels. Amounts over 500 milligrams daily may cause liver damage if taken for prolonged periods.

Vitamin B₅ (Pantothenic Acid)

Known as "the anti-stress vitamin," pantothenic acid plays a role in the production of the adrenal hormones and the formation of antibodies, aids in vitamin utilization, and helps to convert fats, carbohydrates, and proteins into energy. It is required by all cells in the body and is concentrated in the organs. It is also involved in the production of neurotransmitters. This vitamin is an essential element of coenzyme A, a vital body chemical involved in many necessary metabolic functions. Pantothenic acid is also a stamina enhancer and prevents certain forms of anemia. It is needed for normal functioning of the gastrointestinal tract and may be helpful in treating depression and anxiety. A deficiency of pantothenic acid may cause fatigue, headache, nausea, and tingling in the hands. Pantothenic acid is also needed for proper functioning of the adrenal glands.

SOURCES The following foods contain pantothenic acid: beef, brewer's yeast, eggs, fresh vegetables, kidney, legumes, liver, mushrooms, nuts, pork, royal jelly, saltwater fish, torula yeast, whole rye flour, and whole wheat.

Vitamin B₆ (Pyridoxine)

Pyridoxine is involved in more bodily functions than almost any other single nutrient. It affects both physical and mental health. It is beneficial if you suffer from water retention, and is necessary for

35

the production of hydrochloric acid and the absorption of fats and protein. Pyridoxine also aids in maintaining sodium and potassium balance, and promotes red blood cell formation. It is required by the nervous system and is needed for normal brain function and for the synthesis of the nucleic acids RNA and DNA, which contain the genetic instructions for the reproduction of all cells and for normal cellular growth. It activates many enzymes and aids in the absorption of vitamin B_{12}, in immune system function, and in antibody production.

Vitamin B_6 plays a role in cancer immunity and aids in the prevention of arteriosclerosis. It inhibits the formation of a toxic chemical called homocysteine, which attacks the heart muscle and allows the deposition of cholesterol around the heart muscle. Pyridoxine acts as a mild diuretic, reducing the symptoms of premenstrual syndrome, and it may be useful in preventing oxalate kidney stones as well. It is helpful in the treatment of allergies, arthritis, and asthma.

A deficiency of vitamin B_6 can result in anemia, convulsions, headaches, nausea, flaky skin, a sore tongue, and vomiting. Other possible signs of deficiency include acne, anorexia, arthritis, conjunctivitis, cracks or sores on the mouth and lips, depression, dizziness, fatigue, hyperirritability, impaired wound healing, inflammation of the mouth and gums, learning difficulties, impaired memory or memory loss, hair loss, hearing problems, numbness, oily facial skin, stunted growth, and tingling sensations. Carpal tunnel syndrome has been linked to a deficiency of vitamin B_6 as well.

SOURCES All foods contain some vitamin B_6; however, the following foods have the highest amounts: brewer's yeast, carrots, chicken, eggs, fish, meat, peas, spinach, sunflower seeds, walnuts, and wheat germ. Other sources include avocado, bananas, beans, blackstrap molasses, broccoli, brown rice and other whole grains, cabbage, cantaloupe, corn, dulse, plantains, potatoes, rice bran, soybeans, and tempeh. Herbs that contain vitamin B_6 include alfalfa, catnip, and oat straw.

COMMENTS Antidepressants, estrogen therapy, and oral contraceptives may increase the need for vitamin B_6. Diuretics and cortisone drugs block the absorption of this vitamin by the body. Prolonged use of high doses of vitamin B_6 (over 1,000 milligrams per day) can be toxic, and may result in nerve damage and loss of coordination.

Vitamin B_{12} (Cyanocobalamin)

Vitamin B_{12} is needed to prevent anemia. It aids folic acid in regulating the formation of red blood cells, and helps in the utilization of iron. This vitamin is also required for proper digestion, absorption of foods, the synthesis of protein, and the metabolism of carbohydrates and fats. It aids in cell formation and cellular longevity. In addition, vitamin B_{12} prevents nerve damage, maintains fertility, and promotes normal growth and development by maintaining the fatty sheaths that cover and protect nerve endings. Vitamin B_{12} is linked to the production of acetylcholine, a neurotransmitter that assists memory and learning. Vitamin B_{12} supplementation has been shown to enhance sleep patterns, allowing for more restful and refreshing sleep.

A vitamin B_{12} deficiency can be caused by malabsorption, which is most common in elderly people and in those with digestive disorders. Deficiency can cause abnormal gait, bone loss, chronic fatigue, constipation, depression, digestive disorders, dizziness, drowsiness, enlargement of the liver, eye disorders, hallucinations, headaches (including migraines), inflammation of the tongue, irritability, labored breathing, memory loss, moodiness, nervousness, neurological damage, palpitations, pernicious anemia, ringing in the ears, and spinal cord degeneration. Strict vegetarians must remember that they require vitamin B_{12} supplementation, as this vitamin is found almost exclusively in animal tissues. Although people adopting a strictly vegetarian diet may not see any signs of the deficiency for some time—the body can store up to five years' worth of vitamin B_{12}—signs will eventually develop.

SOURCES The largest amounts of vitamin B_{12} are found in brewer's yeast, clams, eggs, herring, kidney, liver, mackerel, milk and dairy products, and seafood. Vitamin B_{12} is not found in many vegetables; it is available only from sea vegetables, such as dulse, kelp, kombu, and nori, and soybeans and soy products. It is also present in the herbs alfalfa, bladderwrack, and hops.

COMMENTS Anti-gout medications, anticoagulant drugs, and potassium supplements may block the absorption of vitamin B_{12} from the digestive tract. Taking vitamin B_{12} in sublingual tablets, which are dissolved under the tongue rather than swallowed, can be a good option for those who have difficulty absorbing this vitamin. *Intrinsic factor* is a protein produced in the gastrointestinal tract that is necessary for absorption of vitamin B_{12}. People who lack intrinsic factor must use a sublingual form for absorption.

Biotin

Biotin aids in cell growth; in fatty acid production; in the metabolism of carbohydrates, fats, and proteins; and in the utilization of the other B-complex vitamins. Sufficient quantities are needed for healthy hair and skin. One hundred milligrams of biotin daily may prevent hair loss in some men. Biotin also promotes healthy sweat glands, nerve tissue, and bone marrow. In addition, it helps to relieve muscle pain.

In infants, a condition called seborrheic dermatitis, or cradle cap, which is characterized by a dry, scaly scalp, may occur as a result of biotin deficiency. In adults, deficiency of this B vitamin is rare because it can be produced in the intestines from foods such as those mentioned below. However, if a deficiency does occur, it can cause anemia, depression, hair loss, high blood sugar, inflammation or pallor of the skin and mucous membranes, insomnia, loss of appetite, muscular pain, nausea, and soreness of the tongue.

SOURCES Biotin is found in brewer's yeast, cooked egg yolks, meat, milk, poultry, saltwater fish, soybeans, and whole grains.

COMMENTS Raw egg whites contain a protein called avidin, which combines with biotin in the intestinal tract and depletes the body of this needed nutrient. Fats and oils that have been subjected to heat or exposed to the air for any length of time inhibit biotin absorption. Antibiotics, sulfa drugs, and saccharin also threaten the availability of biotin.

Choline

Choline is needed for the proper transmission of nerve impulses from the brain through the central nervous system, as well as for gallbladder regulation, liver function, and lecithin formation. It aids in hormone production and minimizes excess fat in the liver because it aids in fat and cholesterol metabolism. Without choline, brain function and memory are impaired. Choline is beneficial for disorders of the nervous system such as Parkinson's disease and tardive dyskinesia. A deficiency may result in fatty buildup in the liver, as well as in cardiac symptoms, gastric ulcers, high blood pressure, an inability to digest fats, kidney and liver impairment, and stunted growth. Research in the last decade indicates that choline plays an important role in cardiovascular health, as well as in reproduction and fetal development. One study showed a need for choline for both prevention and treatment of arteriosclerosis and the metabolism of homocysteine.

SOURCES The following foods contain significant amounts of choline: egg yolks, lecithin (about 13 percent choline by weight), legumes, meat, milk, soybeans, and whole-grain cereals.

Folate

Also known as folacin, folic acid, or pteroylglutamic acid (PGA), folate is considered a brain food, and is needed for energy production and the formation of red blood cells. It also strengthens immunity by aiding in the proper formation and functioning of white blood cells. Because it functions as a coenzyme in DNA and RNA synthesis, it is important for healthy cell division and replication. It is involved in protein metabolism and has been used in the prevention and treatment of folic acid anemia. This nutrient may also help depression and anxiety, and may be effective in the treatment of uterine cervical dysplasia.

Folate may be the most important nutrient in regulating homocysteine levels. Homocysteine is an amino acid that is naturally formed in the body as the result of the breakdown of another amino acid, methionine. In recent years, high levels of homocysteine have been found to be associated with an increased risk of atherosclerosis (hardening of the arteries due to the accumulation of fatty plaques). Normally, homocysteine is converted to other, non-harmful amino acids in the body. In order for this conversion to take place as it should, the body needs an adequate supply of folate, as well as of vitamins B_6 and B_{12}. Homocysteine levels in red blood cells have been shown to have an inverse relationship to levels of these three important B vitamins—that is, the lower the levels of these vitamins, the higher the level of homocysteine.

Folate is very important in pregnancy. It helps to regulate embryonic and fetal nerve cell formation, which is vital for normal development. Studies have shown that a daily intake of 400 micrograms of folate in early pregnancy may prevent the vast majority of neural tube defects, such as spina bifida and anencephaly. It may also help to prevent premature birth. To be effective, this regimen must begin *before* conception and continue for at least the first three months of pregnancy; if a woman waits until she knows she is pregnant, it may be too late, because critical events in fetal development occur during the first six weeks of pregnancy—before many women know that they have conceived. This is why many experts recommend that every woman of childbearing age take a folate supplement daily as a matter of course. Folate works best when combined with vitamin B_{12} and vitamin C.

A sore, red tongue is one sign of folate deficiency. Other possible signs include anemia, apathy, digestive disturbances, fatigue, graying hair, growth impairment, insomnia, labored breathing, memory problems, paranoia, weakness, and birth defects in one's offspring. Folate deficiency may be caused by inadequate consumption of fresh fruits and vegetables; consumption of only cooked or microwaved vegetables (cooking destroys folate); and malabsorption problems.

SOURCES The following foods contain significant quantities of folate: asparagus, barley, beef, bran, brewer's yeast, brown rice, cheese, chicken, dates, green leafy vegetables, lamb, legumes, lentils, liver, milk, mushrooms, oranges, split peas, pork, root vegetables, salmon, tuna, wheat germ, whole grains, and whole wheat.

COMMENTS Oral contraceptives may increase the need for folate. Alcohol also can act as an enemy to folate absorption.

CAUTIONS Do not take high doses of folate for extended periods if you have a hormone-related cancer or seizure disorder.

Inositol

Inositol is vital for hair growth. This vitamin has a calming effect and helps to reduce cholesterol levels. It helps prevent hardening of the arteries and is important in the formation of lecithin and the metabolism of fat and cholesterol. It also helps remove fats from the liver. Deficiency can lead to arteriosclerosis, constipation, hair loss, high blood cholesterol, irritability, mood swings, and skin eruptions. Research has also shown that high doses of inositol may help in the treatment of depression, obsessive-compulsive disorder, and anxiety disorders, without the side effects of prescription medications.

SOURCES Inositol is found in brewer's yeast, fruits, lecithin, legumes, meats, milk, unrefined molasses, raisins, vegetables, and whole grains.

COMMENTS The consumption of large amounts of caffeine may cause a shortage of inositol in the body.

Para-Aminobenzoic Acid (PABA)

PABA is one of the basic constituents of folate and also helps in the assimilation of pantothenic acid. PABA can be converted into folate by intestinal bacteria. This antioxidant helps protect against sunburn (through the absorption of ultraviolet-B [UVB] radiation) and, consequently, skin cancer; acts as a coenzyme in the breakdown and utilization of protein; and assists in the formation of red blood cells. PABA also aids in the maintenance of healthy intestinal flora. Supplementing the diet with PABA may restore gray hair to its original color if the graying was caused by stress or a nutritional deficiency. Other benefits of PABA include protection against secondhand smoke, ozone, and other air pollutants; reduced inflammation in arthritis; and enhanced flexibility.

A deficiency of PABA may lead to depression, fatigue, gastrointestinal disorders, graying of the hair, irritability, nervousness, and patchy areas of white skin.

SOURCES Foods that contain PABA include kidney, liver, molasses, mushrooms, spinach, and whole grains.

COMMENTS Sulfa drugs may cause a deficiency of PABA.

Vitamin C (Ascorbic Acid)

Vitamin C is an antioxidant that is required for at least 300 metabolic functions in the body, including tissue growth and repair, adrenal gland function, and healthy gums. It also aids in the production of anti-stress hormones and interferon, an important immune-system protein, and is needed for the metabolism of folic acid, tyrosine, and phenylalanine. Studies have shown that taking vitamin C can reduce symptoms of asthma. It protects against the harmful effects of pollution, helps to prevent cancer, protects against infection, and enhances immunity. Vitamin C increases the absorption of iron. It can combine with toxic substances, such as certain heavy metals, and render them harmless so that they can be eliminated from the body. Even the venom of a black widow spider may be rendered harmless with the administration of very large doses of vitamin C. This vitamin also may reduce levels of low-density lipoproteins (LDL, the so-called "bad cholesterol"), while increasing levels of high-density lipoproteins (HDL, or "good cholesterol"), as well as lowering high blood pressure and helping to prevent atherosclerosis. Essential in the formation of collagen, vitamin C protects against abnormal blood clotting and bruising, may reduce the risk of cataracts, and promotes the healing of wounds and burns.

Vitamin C works synergistically with both vitamin E and beta-carotene—that is, when these vitamins work together, they have an effect even greater than the sum of their individual effects, and taking them together may counter potential adverse effects of taking these vitamins alone. Vitamin E scavenges for dangerous free radicals in cell membranes, while vitamin C attacks free radicals in biologic fluids. These vitamins reinforce and extend each other's antioxidant activity.

Because the body cannot manufacture vitamin C, it must be obtained through the diet or in the form of supplements. Unfortunately, most of the vitamin C consumed in the diet is lost in the urine. If larger amounts of vitamin C are required due to serious illness, such as cancer, it is more effective to take vitamin C intravenously, under the advisement and supervision of a physician, than it is to take high doses orally.

Scurvy is a disease caused by vitamin C deficiency. It is characterized by poor wound healing, soft and spongy bleeding gums, edema, extreme weakness, and "pinpoint" hemorrhages under the skin. Fortunately, this condition is rare in Western societies. More common are signs of lesser degrees of deficiency, including gums that bleed when brushed; increased susceptibility to infection, especially colds and bronchial infections; joint pains; lack of energy; poor digestion; prolonged wound healing time; a tendency to bruise easily; and tooth loss.

SOURCES Vitamin C is found in berries, citrus fruits, and green vegetables. Good sources include asparagus, avocados, beet greens, black currants, broccoli, Brussels sprouts, cantaloupe, collards, dandelion greens, dulse, grapefruit, kale, lemons, mangos, mustard greens, onions, oranges, papayas, green peas, sweet peppers, persimmons, pineapple, radishes, rose hips, spinach, strawberries, Swiss chard, tomatoes, turnip greens, and watercress. Herbs that contain vitamin C include alfalfa, burdock root, cayenne, chickweed, eyebright, fennel seed, fenugreek, hops, horsetail, kelp, peppermint, mullein, nettle, oat straw, paprika, parsley, pine needle, plantain, raspberry leaf, red clover, rose hips, skullcap, violet leaves, yarrow, and yellow dock.

COMMENTS Alcohol, analgesics, antidepressants, anticoagulants, oral contraceptives, and steroids may reduce levels of vitamin C in the body. Smoking causes a serious depletion of vitamin C.

Diabetes medications such as chlorpropamide (Diabinese) and sulfa drugs may not be as effective if taken with vitamin C. Tak-

43

ing high doses of vitamin C may cause a false-negative reading in tests for blood in the stool.

For maximum effectiveness, supplemental vitamin C should be taken in divided doses, twice daily. Esterified vitamin C (Ester-C) is a remarkably effective form of vitamin C, especially for those suffering from chronic illnesses such as cancer and AIDS. It is created by having the vitamin C react with a necessary mineral, such as calcium, magnesium, potassium, sodium, or zinc. This results in a form of the vitamin that is nonacidic and that contains vitamin C metabolites identical to those produced by the body. Esterified vitamin C enters the bloodstream and tissues four times faster than standard forms of vitamin C because it moves into the blood cells more efficiently and also stays in the body tissues longer. The levels of vitamin C in white blood cells achieved by taking esterified vitamin C are four times higher than those achieved with standard vitamin C. Further, only one-third as much is lost through excretion in the urine. A variety of manufacturers produce supplements containing Ester-C, either by itself or in combination with other valuable nutrients, including the antioxidants Pycnogenol and proanthocyanidins, and the herbs echinacea and garlic.

CAUTIONS If aspirin and standard vitamin C (ascorbic acid) are taken together in large doses, stomach irritation can occur, possibly leading to ulcers. If you take aspirin regularly, use an esterified form of vitamin C, and take it separately from the aspirin.

If you are pregnant, do not take more than 5,000 milligrams of vitamin C daily. A developing infant may become dependent on this supplement and develop scurvy when deprived of the accustomed megadoses after birth.

Avoid using chewable vitamin C supplements, as these can damage tooth enamel.

Vitamin D

Vitamin D, a fat-soluble vitamin that has properties of both a vitamin and a hormone, is required for the absorption and utilization of calcium and phosphorus. It is necessary for growth, and is especially important for the normal growth and development of bones and teeth in children. It protects against muscle weakness and is involved in regulation of the heartbeat. It is also important in the prevention and treatment of breast and colon cancer, osteoarthritis, osteoporosis, and hypocalcemia, enhances immunity, and is necessary for thyroid function and normal blood clotting.

There are several forms of vitamin D, including vitamin D_2 (ergocaliciferol), which comes from food sources; vitamin D_3 (cholecalciferol), which is synthesized in the skin in response to exposure to the sun's ultraviolet rays; and a synthetic form identified as vitamin D_5. Of the three, vitamin D_3 is considered the natural form of vitamin D and is the most active.

The form of vitamin D that we get from food or supplements is not fully active. It requires conversion by the liver, and then by the kidneys, before it becomes fully active. This is why people with liver or kidney disorders are at a higher risk for osteoporosis. When the skin is exposed to the sun's ultraviolet rays, a cholesterol compound in the skin is transformed into a precursor of vitamin D. Exposing the face and arms to the sun for fifteen minutes three times a week is an effective way to ensure adequate amounts of vitamin D in the body. However, researchers have learned that people living in the upper third of the continental United States cannot produce adequate amounts of vitamin D from exposure to the limited available sunlight during the winter months.

45

Severe deficiency of vitamin D can cause rickets in children and osteomalacia, a similar disorder, in adults. Lesser degrees of deficiency may be characterized by loss of appetite, a burning sensation in the mouth and throat, diarrhea, insomnia, visual problems, and weight loss. In a study reported in *The New England Journal of Medicine,* there are indications that vitamin D deficiency is much more widespread than previously thought, especially in older adults. In a group of people of whom few had risk factors for vitamin D deficiency, 57 percent were found to have below-normal levels of vitamin D. Sixty-seven percent of those reporting a vitamin D intake below the RDI had deficiencies categorized as moderate to severe.

SOURCES Fish liver oils, fatty saltwater fish, dairy products, and eggs all contain vitamin D. It is found in butter, cod liver oil, dandelion greens, egg yolks, halibut, liver, milk, oatmeal, salmon, sardines, sweet potatoes, tuna, and vegetable oils. Vitamin D is also formed by the body in response to the action of sunlight on the skin. Herbs that contain vitamin D include alfalfa, horsetail, nettle, and parsley.

COMMENTS Intestinal disorders and liver and gallbladder malfunctions interfere with the absorption of vitamin D. Some cholesterol-lowering drugs, antacids, mineral oil, and steroid hormones such as cortisone also interfere with absorption. Thiazide diuretics such as chlorothiazide (Diuril) and hydrochlorothiazide (Esidrix, HydroDIURIL, Oretic) disturb the body's calcium/vitamin D ratio. Taking excessive amounts of vitamin D (over 1,000 international units) daily may cause a decrease in bone mass.

CAUTIONS Do not take vitamin D without calcium. Toxicity may result from taking excessive amounts of supplemental vitamin D.

Vitamin E

Vitamin E is an antioxidant that is important in the prevention of cancer and cardiovascular disease. It improves circulation, is necessary for tissue repair, and is useful in treating premenstrual syndrome and fibrocystic disease of the breast. It promotes normal blood clotting and healing, reduces scarring from some wounds, reduces blood pressure, aids in preventing cataracts, improves athletic performance, and relaxes leg cramps. Vitamin E can enhance sperm production in some men. It also maintains healthy nerves and muscles while strengthening capillary walls. In addition, it promotes healthy skin and hair, and helps to prevent anemia and retrolental fibroplasia, an eye disorder that can affect premature infants. A 1998 study by the National Cancer Institute found that long-term use of vitamin E substantially reduced prostate cancer risk in smokers. Other studies suggest that this vitamin may slow the progression of Alzheimer's disease. Thus far, vitamin E has been shown to protect against approximately eighty diseases.

As an antioxidant, vitamin E prevents cell damage by inhibiting the oxidation of lipids (fats) and the formation of free radicals. It protects other fat-soluble vitamins from destruction by oxygen and aids in the utilization of vitamin A. It retards aging and may prevent age spots as well. Some studies have shown daily use of vitamin E to be more protective than aspirin for prevention of heart attacks, with no harmful side effects. The misuse of aspirin, in contrast, causes or contributes to an estimated 3,000 deaths in the United States each year.

Vitamin E deficiency may result in damage to red blood cells and destruction of nerves. Signs of deficiency can include infertility (in both men and women), menstrual problems, neuromuscular impairment, shortened red blood cell lifespan, spontaneous abortion (miscarriage), and uterine degeneration. Low levels of vitamin E in the body have been linked to both bowel cancer and breast cancer. Epidemiological links have been identified between the increase in the incidence of heart disease and the increasing lack of vitamin E in the American diet due to our reliance on over-processed foods.

Vitamin E is actually a family of eight different but related molecules that fall into two major groups: the tocopherols and the tocotrienols. Within each group, there are alpha, beta, gamma, and delta forms. Of all eight of these molecules, it is the d-alpha-tocopherol form that is the most potent. Natural sources of vitamin E are better than synthetic vitamin E because natural vitamin E is more available for use by the body than the synthetic form. Synthetic vitamin E is only 67 percent as active as the natural form. Read labels closely. The natural form of vitamin E is listed as *d-alpha-tocopherol;* the synthetic form is listed as *dl-alpha-tocopherol* (watch out for the *l* after the *d*). The *dl* form costs only about half as much as the *d* form, but it has significantly less activity, or potency.

SOURCES Vitamin E is found in the following food sources: cold-pressed vegetable oils, dark green leafy vegetables, legumes, nuts, seeds, and whole grains. Significant quantities of this vitamin are also found in brown rice, cornmeal, dulse, eggs, kelp, desiccated liver, milk, oatmeal, organ meats, soybeans, sweet potatoes, watercress, wheat, and wheat germ. Herbs that contain vitamin E include alfalfa, bladderwrack, dandelion, dong quai, flaxseed, nettle, oat straw, raspberry leaf, and rose hips.

COMMENTS The body needs zinc in order to maintain the proper level of vitamin E in the blood. Vitamin E that has oxidized a free radical can be revitalized by vitamin C and enabled to battle additional free radicals, according to Lester Packer, Ph.D., noted researcher and professor of molecular and cell biology at the University of California—Berkeley. Adding vitamin E to fats and oils prevents them from becoming rancid. The oxidation of fats is a key factor in the formation of plaque adhering to blood vessel walls.

If you take both vitamin E and iron supplements, take them at different times of the day. Inorganic forms of iron (such as ferrous sulfate) destroy vitamin E. Organic iron (ferrous gluconate or ferrous fumarate) leaves vitamin E intact.

CAUTIONS If you are taking an anticoagulant medication (blood thinner), do not take more than 1,200 international units of vitamin E daily. If you suffer from diabetes, rheumatic heart disease, or an overactive thyroid, do not take more than the recommended dose. If you have high blood pressure, start with a small amount, such as 200 international units daily, and increase slowly to the desired amount.

Vitamin K

Vitamin K is needed for the production of prothrombin, which is necessary for blood clotting. It is also essential for bone formation and repair; it is necessary for the synthesis of osteocalcin, the protein in bone tissue on which calcium crystallizes. Consequently, it may help prevent osteoporosis.

Vitamin K plays an important role in the intestines and aids in converting glucose into glycogen for storage in the liver, promoting healthy liver function. It may increase resistance to infection in children and help prevent cancers that target the inner linings of the organs. It aids in promoting longevity. A deficiency of this vitamin can cause abnormal and/or internal bleeding.

There are three forms of vitamin K: vitamin K_1 (phylloquinone or phytonactone), which comes from plants; vitamin K_2, a family of substances called menaquinones, which are made by intestinal bacteria; and vitamin K_3 (menadione), which is a synthetic substance.

SOURCES Vitamin K is found in some foods, including asparagus, blackstrap molasses, broccoli, Brussels sprouts, cabbage, cauliflower, dark green leafy vegetables, egg yolks, leaf lettuce, liver, oatmeal, oats, rye, safflower oil, soybeans, wheat, and yogurt. Herbs that can supply vitamin K include alfalfa, green tea, kelp, nettle, oat straw, and shepherd's purse. However, the majority of the body's supply of this vitamin is synthesized by the "friendly" bacteria normally present in the intestines.

COMMENTS Antibiotics increase the need for dietary or supplemental vitamin K. Because vitamin K is synthesized by bacteria in the intestines, taking antibiotics—which kill the bacteria—interferes with this process. Antibiotics also interfere with the absorption of vitamin K.

CAUTIONS Do not take large doses of synthetic vitamin K during the last few weeks of pregnancy. It can result in a toxic reaction in the newborn. If you are taking anticoagulant (blood thinning) drugs, consult with your health care provider before taking any supplemental vitamin K, as it can interfere with the action of these medications. Megadoses of this vitamin can accumulate in the body and cause flushing and sweating.

Bioflavonoids

Although bioflavonoids are not true vitamins in the strictest sense, they are sometimes referred to as vitamin P. Bioflavonoids are essential for the absorption of vitamin C, and the two should be taken together. There are many different bioflavonoids, including citrin, eriodictyol, flavones, hesperetin, hesperidin, quercetin, quercetrin, and rutin. The human body cannot produce bioflavonoids, so they must be supplied in the diet.

Bioflavonoids are used extensively in the treatment of athletic injuries because they relieve pain, bumps, and bruises. They also reduce pain located in the legs or across the back, and lessen symptoms associated with prolonged bleeding and low serum calcium. Bioflavonoids act synergistically with vitamin C to protect and preserve the structure of capillaries. In addition, bioflavonoids have an antibacterial effect and promote circulation, stimulate bile production, lower cholesterol levels, and treat and prevent cataracts. When taken with vitamin C, bioflavonoids also reduce the symptoms of oral herpes.

Quercetin, a bioflavonoid available in supplement form, may effectively treat and prevent asthma symptoms. Activated Quercetin from Source Naturals is a good source of quercetin. It also contains two other ingredients that increase its efficacy: bromelain, an enzyme from pineapple, and vitamin C, in the nonacidic form of magnesium ascorbate. Bromelain and quercetin are synergists, and should be taken in conjunction to enhance absorption.

SOURCES Peppers, buckwheat, black currants, and the white material just beneath the peel of citrus fruits contain bioflavonoids. Sources of bioflavonoids include apricots, blackberries, cherries, grapefruit, grapes, lemons, oranges, plums, prunes, and rose hips. Herbs that contain bioflavonoids include chervil, elderberries, hawthorn berry, horsetail, rose hips, and shepherd's purse.

COMMENTS Extremely high doses may cause diarrhea.

Coenzyme Q$_{10}$

Coenzyme Q$_{10}$ is a vitamin-like substance found in all parts of the body whose actions resemble those of vitamin E. It may be an even more powerful antioxidant. It is also called ubiquinone. There are ten common substances designated coenzyme Qs, but coenzyme Q$_{10}$ is the only one found in human tissue. This substance plays a critical role in the production of energy in every cell of the body. It aids circulation, stimulates the immune system, increases tissue oxygenation, and has vital anti-aging effects. Deficiencies of coenzyme Q$_{10}$ have been linked to periodontal disease, diabetes, and muscular dystrophy.

Research has revealed that supplemental coenzyme Q$_{10}$ has the ability to counter histamine, and therefore is beneficial for people with allergies, asthma, or respiratory disease. It is used by many health care professionals to treat anomalies of mental function such as those associated with schizophrenia and Alzheimer's disease. It is also beneficial in fighting obesity, candidiasis, multiple sclerosis, and diabetes.

Coenzyme Q_{10} appears to be a giant step forward in the treatment and prevention of cardiovascular disease. A six-year study conducted by scientists at the University of Texas found that people being treated for congestive heart failure who took coenzyme Q_{10} in addition to conventional therapy had a 75-percent chance of survival after three years, compared with a 25-percent survival rate for those using conventional therapy alone. In a similar study by the University of Texas and the Center for Adult Diseases in Japan, coenzyme Q_{10} was shown to be able to lower high blood pressure without medication or dietary changes.

In addition to its use in fighting cardiovascular disease, coenzyme Q_{10} has been shown to be effective in reducing mortality in experimental animals afflicted with tumors and leukemia. Some doctors give their patients coenzyme Q_{10} to reduce the side effects of cancer chemotherapy.

Coenzyme Q_{10} is widely used in Japan. More than 12 million people in that country are reportedly taking it at the direction of their physicians for treatment of heart disease (it strengthens the heart muscle) and high blood pressure, and also to enhance the immune system. Research in Japan has shown that coenzyme Q_{10} also protects the stomach lining and duodenum, and may help heal duodenal ulcers.

The amount of coenzyme Q_{10} present in the body declines with age, so it should be supplemented in the diet, especially by people who are over the age of fifty. A sublingual form containing 50 milligrams of this vital nutrient, available from FoodScience Laboratories, is an especially easy to assimilate supplement. Nature's Plus and Carlson Labs both make soft gel-capsules of coenzyme Q_{10} in dosage levels up to 100 milligrams. Oil-based forms are best.

SOURCES Mackerel, salmon, and sardines contain the largest amounts of coenzyme Q_{10}. It is also found in beef, peanuts, and spinach.

COMMENTS Coenzyme Q_{10} is oil soluble and is best absorbed when taken with oily or fatty foods, such as fish. Be cautious when purchasing coenzyme Q_{10}. Not all products offer it in its purest form. Its natural color is dark bright yellow to orange, and it has very little taste in the powdered form. It should be kept away from heat and light. Pure coenzyme Q_{10} is perishable and deteriorates in temperatures above 115°F. A liquid or oil form is preferable. Look for a product that includes a small amount of vitamin E, as this helps to preserve the coenzyme Q_{10}.

THREE

Minerals

INTRODUCTION

Every living cell on this planet depends on minerals for proper function and structure. Minerals are needed for the proper composition of body fluids, the formation of blood and bone, the maintenance of healthy nerve function, and the regulation of muscle tone, including that of the muscles of the cardiovascular system. Like vitamins, minerals function as coenzymes, enabling the body to perform its functions, including energy production, growth, and healing. Because all enzyme activities involve minerals, minerals are essential for the proper utilization of vitamins and other nutrients.

The human body, as all of nature, must maintain its proper chemical balance. This balance depends on the levels of different minerals in the body and especially the ratios of certain mineral levels to one another. The level of each mineral in the body has an effect on every other, so if one is out of balance, all mineral levels are affected. If not corrected, this can start a chain reaction of imbalances that leads to illness.

Minerals are naturally occurring elements found in the earth. Rock formations are made up of mineral salts. Rock and stone are gradually broken down into tiny fragments by erosion, a process that can take literally millions of years. The resulting dust and sand accumulate, forming the basis of soil. The soil is teeming with microbes that utilize these tiny crystals of mineral salts, which are then passed from the soil to plants. The plants are eaten by herbivorous animals. We obtain these minerals by consuming plants or herbivorous animals.

Nutritionally, minerals belong to two groups: bulk minerals (also called macrominerals) and trace minerals (microminerals). Bulk minerals include calcium, magnesium, sodium, potassium, and phosphorus. These are needed in larger amounts than trace minerals. Although only minute quantities of trace minerals are needed, they are nevertheless important for good health. Trace minerals include boron, chromium, copper, germanium, iodine, iron, manganese, molybdenum, selenium, silicon, sulfur, vanadium, and zinc.

Because minerals are stored primarily in the body's bone and muscle tissue, it is possible to develop mineral toxicity if extremely large quantities are consumed. Such situations are rare, however, because toxic levels of minerals generally accumulate only if massive amounts are ingested for a prolonged period of time.

WHAT'S ON THE SHELVES

As with vitamins, it can be difficult, if not impossible, to obtain the amounts of minerals needed for optimum health through diet alone. Mineral supplements can help you to make sure you are getting all the minerals your body requires.

Minerals are often found in multivitamin formulas. Minerals can also be sold as single supplements. These are available in tablet, capsule, powder, and liquid forms. Some are available in chelated form, which means that the minerals are bonded to protein molecules that transport them to the bloodstream and enhance their absorption. When mineral supplements are taken with a meal, they are usually automatically chelated in the stomach during digestion. There is some controversy over which mineral supplements are best, but we prefer the chelated preparations. Our experience with the various chelated formulas available has shown that, in general, arginate forms of minerals make the most effective supplements.

Once a mineral is absorbed, it must be carried by the blood to the cells and then transported across the cell membranes in a form that can be utilized by the cells. After minerals enter the body, they compete with one another for absorption. For example, too much zinc can deplete the body of copper; excessive calcium intake can affect magnesium absorption. Consequently, supplemental minerals should always be taken in balanced amounts. Otherwise, they will not be effective and may even be harmful. The absorption of minerals can also be affected by the use of fiber supplements. Fiber decreases the body's absorption of minerals. Therefore, supplemental fiber and minerals should be taken at different times.

THE ABC'S OF MINERALS

Boron

55

Boron is needed in trace amounts for healthy bones and muscle growth because it assists in the production of natural steroid compounds within the body. It is also necessary for the metabolism of calcium, phosphorus, and magnesium. It enhances brain function, promotes alertness, and plays a role in how the body utilizes energy from fats and sugars. Most people are not deficient in boron. However, elderly people usually benefit from taking a supplement of 2 to 3 milligrams daily because they have greater problems with calcium absorption. Boron deficiency accentuates vitamin D deficiency.

Boron helps to prevent postmenopausal osteoporosis and build muscle. A study conducted by the U.S. Department of Agriculture indicated that within eight days of supplementing their daily diet with 3 milligrams of boron, a test group of postmenopausal women lost 40 percent less calcium, one-third less magnesium, and slightly less phosphorus through their urine than they had before beginning boron supplementation.

SOURCES Boron is found in apples, carrots, grapes, dark green leafy vegetables, raw nuts, pears, and whole grains.

CAUTIONS Do not take more than 3 to 6 milligrams unless prescribed.

Calcium

Calcium is vital for the formation of strong bones and teeth and for the maintenance of healthy gums. It is also important in the maintenance of a regular heartbeat and in the transmission of nerve impulses. Calcium lowers cholesterol levels and helps prevent cardiovascular disease. It is needed for muscular growth and contraction, and for the prevention of muscle cramps. It may increase the rate of bone growth and bone mineral density in children. This important mineral is also essential in blood clotting and helps prevent cancer. It may lower blood pressure and prevent bone loss associated with osteoporosis as well. Calcium provides energy and participates in the protein structuring of RNA and DNA. It is also involved in the activation of several enzymes, including lipase, which breaks down fats for utilization by the body. In addition, calcium maintains proper cell membrane permeability, aids in neuromuscular activity, helps to keep the skin healthy, and protects against the development of preeclampsia during pregnancy, the number one cause of maternal death. If high blood pressure develops due to pregnancy, it can be reduced by calcium intake.

Calcium protects the bones and teeth from lead by inhibiting absorption of this toxic metal. If there is a calcium deficiency, lead can be absorbed by the body and deposited in the teeth and bones.

Calcium deficiency can lead to the following problems: aching joints, brittle nails, eczema, elevated blood cholesterol, heart palpitations, hypertension (high blood pressure), insomnia, muscle cramps, nervousness, numbness in the arms and/or legs, a pasty complexion, rheumatoid arthritis, rickets, and tooth decay. Deficiencies of calcium are also associated with cognitive impairment, convulsions, depression, delusions, and hyperactivity.

SOURCES Calcium is found in dairy foods, salmon (with bones), sardines, seafood, and dark green leafy vegetables. Food sources include almonds, asparagus, blackstrap molasses, brewer's yeast, broccoli, buttermilk, cabbage, carob, cheese, collards, dandelion greens, dulse, figs, filberts, goat's milk, kale, kelp, milk, mustard greens, oats, prunes, sesame seeds, soybeans, tofu, turnip greens, watercress, whey, and yogurt. Herbs that contain calcium include alfalfa, burdock root, cayenne, chamomile, chickweed, chicory, dandelion, eyebright, fennel seed, fenugreek, flaxseed, hops, horsetail, kelp, lemongrass, mullein, nettle, oat straw, paprika, parsley, peppermint, plantain, raspberry leaves, red clover, rose hips, shepherd's purse, violet leaves, yarrow, and yellow dock.

COMMENTS The amino acid lysine is needed for calcium absorption. Food sources of lysine include cheese, eggs, fish, lima beans, milk, potatoes, red meat, soy products, and brewer's yeast. Lysine is also available in supplement form.

Female athletes and menopausal women need greater amounts of calcium than other women because their estrogen levels are lower. Estrogen protects the skeletal system by promoting the deposition of calcium in bone.

Heavy exercising hinders calcium uptake, but moderate exercise promotes it. Insufficient vitamin D intake, or the ingestion of excessive amounts of phosphorus and magnesium, also hinders the uptake of calcium.

If calcium is taken with iron, they bind together, preventing the optimal absorption of both minerals. It is therefore best to take calcium and iron at different times. Too much calcium can interfere with the absorption of zinc, and excess zinc can interfere with calcium absorption (especially if calcium intake is low). For most people, the best ratio between supplemental calcium and zinc is up to 2,500 milligrams of calcium with 50 milligrams of zinc daily. A hair analysis can determine the levels of these and other minerals in the body.

A diet that is high in protein, fat, and/or sugar affects calcium uptake. The average American diet of meats, refined grains, and soft drinks (which are high in phosphorus) leads to increased excretion of calcium. Consuming alcoholic beverages, coffee, junk foods, excess salt, and/or white flour also leads to the loss of calcium by the body. A diet based on foods such as vegetables, fruits, and whole grains, which contain significant amounts of calcium but lower amounts of phosphorus, is preferable.

Oxalic acid (found in almonds, beet greens, cashews, chard, cocoa, kale, rhubarb, soybeans, and spinach) interferes with calcium absorption by binding with it in the intestines and producing insoluble salts that cannot be absorbed. Normal consumption of foods containing oxalic acid should not pose a problem, but overindulgence in these foods inhibits the absorption of calcium. Oxalic acid can also combine with calcium to form calcium-oxalate kidney stones. Studies have shown, however, that taking magnesium and potassium supplements can prevent the formation of this type of stone.

Calcium supplements are more effective when taken in smaller doses spread throughout the day and before bedtime. This mineral works less effectively when taken in a single megadose. Most experts agree that no more than 500 milligrams should be taken at one time, as this is the maximum amount the body can absorb in one dose. However, because calcium also promotes a sound sleep when taken at night, and because a high-fiber diet can interfere with calcium absorption, some recommend taking a single dose at bedtime.

Some vitamin companies use a compound called D_1-calcium-phosphate in their products. This form of calcium is insoluble and interferes with the absorption of the nutrients in a multinutrient supplement. Antacids such as Tums are not recommended as a source of calcium. While they do contain calcium, if taken in sufficient quantities to serve as a source of this mineral, they would also neutralize the stomach acid needed for calcium absorption. Additionally, a significant percentage (estimates range from 20 to 40 percent) of people over the age of sixty may have a condition called atrophic gastritis. This is a chronic inflammation of the stomach, and it reduces the ability to break down the calcium carbonate contained in Tums.

Calcium Absorption Formula from A. Vogel Homeopathic is a sublingual calcium supplement that is especially effective for growing children, older adults, pregnant women, and anyone who has difficulty swallowing pills.

CAUTIONS Calcium may interfere with the effects of verapamil (Calan, Isoptin, Verelan), a calcium channel blocker sometimes prescribed for heart problems and high blood pressure. Calcium can also interfere with the effectiveness of tetracycline, thyroid hormone, certain anticonvulsants, and steroids. Consult your health care provider before taking supplemental calcium if you must take any of these drugs.

Phenobarbital and diuretics may cause a deficiency of calcium. Although several major studies have shown that added calcium in the diet does not appear to increase the risk for either a first or repeat attack of kidney stones, persons with a history of kidney stones or kidney disease should not take calcium supplements except on the advice of a physician. The maximum safe dosage of supplemental calcium is now placed at 2,500 milligrams per day.

Chromium

59

Because it is involved in the metabolism of glucose, chromium (sometimes also called glucose tolerance factor or GTF) is needed for energy. It is also vital in the synthesis of cholesterol, fats, and proteins. This essential mineral maintains stable blood sugar levels through proper insulin utilization, and can be helpful both for people with diabetes and those with hypoglycemia. Studies have shown that low plasma chromium levels can be an indication of coronary artery disease. Additional chromium is needed during pregnancy because the developing fetus increases demand for this mineral. Chromium supplements can help an expectant mother maintain healthy blood sugar levels during pregnancy.

The average American diet is chromium deficient. Only one in ten Americans has an adequate amount of chromium in his or her diet. There are five main reasons for this: The form of chromium in many foods is not easily absorbed; not enough foods containing chromium are consumed; much of the chromium content is lost during processing; many people do not like the foods that are the best sources of chromium; and high quantities of sugar in the diet cause a loss of chromium from the body. Researchers estimate that two out of every three Americans are hypoglycemic, prehypoglycemic, or diabetic. The ability to maintain normal blood sugar levels is jeopardized by the lack of chromium in our soil and water supply and by a diet high in refined white sugar, flour, and junk foods.

A deficiency of chromium can lead to anxiety, fatigue, glucose intolerance (particularly in people with diabetes), inadequate metabolism of amino acids, and an increased risk of arteriosclerosis. Excessive intake (the level depends upon individual tolerance) can lead to chromium toxicity, which has been associated with dermatitis, gastrointestinal ulcers, and kidney and liver impairment.

Supplemental chromium is best absorbed by the body when it is taken in a form called *chromium picolinate* (chromium chelated with picolinate, a naturally occurring amino acid metabolite). Picolinate enables chromium to readily enter into the body's cells, where the mineral can then help insulin do its job much more effectively. Chromium picolinate has been used successfully to control blood cholesterol and blood glucose levels. It also promotes the loss of fat and an increase in lean muscle tissue. Studies show it may increase longevity and help to fight osteoporosis. Chromium polynicotinate (chromium bonded to niacin) is an effective form of this mineral as well.

SOURCES Chromium is found in the following food sources: beer, brewer's yeast, brown rice, cheese, meat, and whole grains. It may also be found in dried beans, blackstrap molasses, calf liver, chicken, corn and corn oil, dairy products, dried liver, dulse, eggs, mushrooms, and potatoes. Herbs that contain chromium include catnip, horsetail, licorice, nettle, oat straw, red clover, sarsaparilla, wild yam, and yarrow.

COMMENTS Active, athletic individuals—people who engage in vigorous aerobic activities and consume higher amounts of carbohydrates than the general population—have higher chromium requirements than nonathletes. Chromium levels start to decrease as we age, starting in our early forties. Some smaller studies have confirmed that added chromium in the diet can reduce total body fat and increase the percentage of muscle.

CAUTIONS If you have insulin-dependent diabetes, you should not use chromium unless it is prescribed by your health care practitioner. Chromium supplements can make insulin function more effectively and, in effect, reduce insulin requirements. People with diabetes therefore have to monitor their blood sugar levels very carefully when using chromium. Chromium requirements differ from person to person; consult your health care provider to determine the correct amount of this mineral for you.

Some people experience lightheadedness or a slight skin rash when taking chromium. If you feel lightheaded, stop taking the supplement and consult your health care provider. If you develop a rash, either try switching brands or discontinue use.

Copper

Among its many functions, copper aids in the formation of bone, hemoglobin, and red blood cells, and works in balance with zinc and vitamin C to form elastin, an important skin protein. It is involved in the healing process, energy production, hair and skin coloring, and taste sensitivity. This mineral is also needed for healthy nerves and joints.

One of the early signs of copper deficiency is osteoporosis. Copper is essential for the formation of collagen, one of the fundamental proteins making up bones, skin, and connective tissue. Other possible signs of copper deficiency include anemia, baldness, diarrhea, general weakness, impaired respiratory function, and skin sores. A lack of copper can also lead to increased blood fat levels.

Excessive intake of copper can lead to toxicity, which has been associated with depression, irritability, nausea and vomiting, nervousness, and joint and muscle pain. Ingesting a quantity as small as 10 milligrams usually causes nausea. Sixty milligrams generally results in vomiting, and just 3.5 grams (3,500 milligrams) can be fatal. Children can be affected at much smaller dosage levels.

SOURCES Besides its use in cookware and plumbing, copper is also widely distributed in foods. Food sources include almonds, avocados, barley, beans, beets, blackstrap molasses, broccoli, garlic, lentils, liver, mushrooms, nuts, oats, oranges, pecans, radishes, raisins, salmon, seafood, soybeans, and green leafy vegetables.

COMMENTS The level of copper in the body is related to the levels of zinc and vitamin C. Copper levels are reduced if large amounts of zinc or vitamin C are consumed. If copper intake is too high, levels of vitamin C and zinc drop.

The consumption of high amounts of fructose (fruit sugar) can make a copper deficiency significantly worse. In a study conducted by the U.S. Department of Agriculture, people who obtained 20 percent of their daily calories from fructose showed decreased levels of red blood cell superoxide dismutase (SOD), a copper-dependent enzyme critical to antioxidant protection within the red blood cells.

CAUTIONS Excessive copper in the body can promote destruction of eye tissue through oxidation. Persons with eye problems should be especially careful to balance their intake of copper with that of iron, zinc, and calcium.

Germanium

Germanium improves cellular oxygenation. This helps to fight pain, keep the immune system functioning properly, and rid the body of toxins and poisons. Researchers have shown that consuming foods containing organic germanium is an effective way to increase tissue oxygenation, because, like hemoglobin, germanium acts as a carrier of oxygen to the cells. A Japanese scientist, Kazuhiko Asai, found that an intake of 100 to 300 milligrams of germanium per day improved many illnesses, including rheumatoid arthritis, food allergies, elevated cholesterol, candidiasis, chronic viral infections, cancer, and AIDS.

SOURCES Germanium is found in all organic material, of both plant and animal origin. The following foods contain the greatest concentrations of germanium: broccoli, celery, garlic, shiitake mushrooms, milk, onions, rhubarb, sauerkraut, tomato juice, and the herbs aloe vera, comfrey, ginseng, and suma.

COMMENTS Germanium is best obtained through the diet.

CAUTIONS Although it is rare, some individuals may develop kidney problems or have a toxic reaction to this mineral if they take it in excessive amounts.

Iodine

Needed only in trace amounts, iodine helps to metabolize excess fat and is important for physical and mental development. It is also needed for a healthy thyroid gland and for the prevention of goiter. Iodine deficiency in children may result in mental retardation. In addition, iodine deficiency has been linked to breast cancer and is associated with fatigue, neonatal hypothyroidism, and weight gain. Excessive iodine intake (sometimes as little as 750 micrograms daily) may inhibit the secretion of thyroid hormone and can produce a metallic taste and sores in the mouth, swollen salivary glands, diarrhea, and vomiting.

SOURCES Foods that are high in iodine include dairy products (from cattle fed iodine-supplemented feed and salt licks), iodized salt, seafood, saltwater fish, and kelp. It may also be found in asparagus, dulse, garlic, lima beans, mushrooms, sea salt (which provides nature's own balance of minerals), sesame seeds, soybeans, spinach (but *see* Comments, below), summer squash, Swiss chard, and turnip greens.

COMMENTS Some foods block the uptake of iodine into the thyroid gland when eaten raw in large amounts. These include Brussels sprouts, cabbage, cauliflower, kale, peaches, pears, spinach, and turnips. If you have an underactive thyroid, you should limit your consumption of these foods.

Iron

Perhaps the most important of iron's functions in the body is the production of hemoglobin and myoglobin (the form of hemoglobin found in muscle tissue), and the oxygenation of red blood cells. Iron is the mineral found in the largest amounts in the blood.

It is essential for many enzymes, including catalase, and is important for growth. Iron is also required for a healthy immune system and for energy production.

Iron deficiency is most often caused by insufficient intake. However, it may result from intestinal bleeding, a diet high in phosphorus, poor digestion, long-term illness, ulcers, prolonged use of antacids, excessive coffee or tea consumption, and other causes. Menstruating women may become iron deficient, especially if they have heavy or prolonged periods and/or short menstrual cycles. In some cases, a deficiency of vitamin B_6 (pyridoxine) or vitamin B_{12} can be the underlying cause of anemia. Strenuous exercise and heavy perspiration deplete iron from the body.

Iron deficiency symptoms include anemia, brittle hair, difficulty swallowing, digestive disturbances, dizziness, fatigue, fragile bones, hair loss, inflammation of the tissues of the mouth, nails that are spoon-shaped or that have ridges running lengthwise, nervousness, obesity, pallor, and slowed mental reactions.

Because iron is stored in the body, excessive iron intake can also cause problems. Too much iron in the tissues and organs leads to the production of free radicals and increases the need for vitamin E. High levels of iron have also been found in association with heart disease and cancer. The buildup of iron in the tissues has been associated with a rare disease known as hemochromatosis, a hereditary disorder of iron metabolism that is found mostly in men and that causes excessive absorption of iron from both foods and supplements, leading to bronze skin pigmentation, arthritis, cirrhosis of the liver, diabetes, and heart disorders.

SOURCES Iron is found in eggs, fish, liver, meat, poultry, green leafy vegetables, whole grains, and enriched breads and cereals. Other food sources include almonds, avocados, beets, blackstrap molasses, brewer's yeast, dates, dulse, kelp, kidney and lima beans, lentils, millet, peaches, pears, dried prunes, pumpkins, raisins, rice and wheat bran, sesame seeds, soybeans, and watercress. Herbs that contain iron include alfalfa, burdock root, catnip, cayenne, chamomile, chickweed, chicory, dandelion, dong quai, eyebright, fennel seed, fenugreek, horsetail, kelp, lemongrass, licorice, milk thistle seed, mullein, nettle, oat straw, paprika, parsley, peppermint, plantain, raspberry leaf, rose hips, sarsaparilla, shepherd's purse, uva ursi, and yellow dock.

COMMENTS Unless you are diagnosed as anemic, you should not take iron supplements. If you take a multivitamin and mineral supplement, choose a product that does not contain iron. If you do need to take iron supplements, do not take them at the same time as vitamin E, and choose an organic form of iron such as ferrous gluconate or ferrous fumarate. Inorganic forms of iron, such as ferrous sulfate, can oxidize vitamin E.

There must be sufficient hydrochloric acid (HCl) present in the stomach in order for iron to be absorbed. Copper, manganese, molybdenum, vitamin A, and the B-complex vitamins are also needed for complete iron absorption. Taking vitamin C can increase iron absorption by as much as 30 percent.

Taking calcium with meals can inhibit the absorption of iron from dietary sources. If you are iron deficient, take calcium supplements at bedtime or at other times when you are not consuming foods containing iron. Excessive amounts of zinc and vitamin E can also interfere with iron absorption. The utilization of iron may be impaired by rheumatoid arthritis and cancer. These diseases can result in anemia despite adequate amounts of iron stored in the liver, spleen, and bone marrow. Iron deficiency is more prevalent in people with candidiasis or chronic herpes infections.

CAUTIONS Do not take iron supplements if you have an infection. Because bacteria require iron for growth, the body "hides" iron in the liver and other storage sites when an infection is present. Taking extra iron at such times encourages the proliferation of bacteria in the body.

Magnesium

Magnesium is a vital catalyst in enzyme activity, especially the activity of those enzymes involved in energy production. It also assists in calcium and potassium uptake. A deficiency of magnesium interferes with the transmission of nerve and muscle impulses, causing irritability and nervousness. Supplementing the diet with magnesium can help prevent depression, dizziness, muscle weakness and twitching, and premenstrual syndrome (PMS), and also aids in maintaining the body's proper pH balance and normal body temperature.

Magnesium is necessary to prevent the calcification of soft tissue. This essential mineral protects the arterial linings from stress caused by sudden blood pressure changes, and plays a role in the formation of bone and in carbohydrate and mineral metabolism. With vitamin B_6 (pyridoxine), magnesium helps to reduce and dissolve calcium phosphate kidney stones, and may prevent calcium-oxalate kidney stones. Research has shown that magnesium may help prevent cardiovascular disease, osteoporosis, and certain forms of cancer, and it may reduce cholesterol levels. It is effective in preventing premature labor and convulsions in pregnant women.

Studies have shown that taking magnesium supplements during pregnancy has a dramatic effect in reducing birth defects. A study reported by the *Journal of the American Medical Association* reported a 70-percent lower incidence of mental retardation in the children of mothers who had taken magnesium supplements during pregnancy. The incidence of cerebral palsy was 90 percent lower.

Possible manifestations of magnesium deficiency include confusion, insomnia, irritability, poor digestion, rapid heartbeat, seizures, and tantrums; often, a magnesium deficiency can be synonymous with diabetes. Magnesium deficiencies are at the root of many cardiovascular problems. Magnesium deficiency may be a major cause of fatal cardiac arrhythmia, hypertension, and sudden cardiac arrest, as well as asthma, chronic fatigue, chronic pain syndromes, depression, insomnia, irritable bowel syndrome, and pulmonary disorders. Research has also shown that magnesium deficiency may contribute to the formation of kidney stones. To test for magnesium deficiency, a procedure called an intracellular (mononuclear cell) magnesium screen should be performed. This is a more sensitive test than the typical serum magnesium screen, and can detect a deficiency with more accuracy. Magnesium screening should be a routine test, as a low magnesium level makes nearly every disease worse. It is particularly important for individuals who have, or who are considered at risk for developing, cardiovascular disease.

SOURCES Magnesium is found in most foods, especially dairy products, fish, meat, and seafood. Other rich food sources include apples, apricots, avocados, bananas, blackstrap molasses, brewer's yeast, brown rice, cantaloupe, dulse, figs, garlic, grapefruit, green leafy vegetables, kelp, lemons, lima beans, millet, nuts, peaches, black-eyed peas, salmon, sesame seeds, soybeans, tofu, torula yeast, watercress, wheat, and whole grains. Herbs that contain magnesium include alfalfa, bladderwrack, catnip, cayenne, chamomile, chickweed, dandelion, eyebright, fennel seed, fenugreek, hops, horsetail, lemongrass, licorice, mullein, nettle, oat straw, paprika, parsley, peppermint, raspberry leaf, red clover, sage, shepherd's purse, yarrow, and yellow dock.

COMMENTS The consumption of alcohol, the use of diuretics, diarrhea, the presence of fluoride, and high levels of zinc and vitamin D all increase the body's need for magnesium.

The consumption of large amounts of fats, cod liver oil, calcium, vitamin D, and protein decrease magnesium absorption. Fat-soluble vitamins also hinder the absorption of magnesium, as do foods high in oxalic acid, such as almonds, chard, cocoa, rhubarb, spinach, and tea.

Manganese

Minute quantities of manganese are needed for protein and fat metabolism, healthy nerves, a healthy immune system, and blood sugar regulation. Manganese is used in energy production and is required for normal bone growth and for reproduction. In addition, it is used in the formation of cartilage and synovial (lubricating) fluid of the joints. It is also necessary for the synthesis of bone.

Manganese is essential for people with iron-deficiency anemias and is needed for the utilization of vitamin B_1 (thiamine) and vitamin E. Manganese works well with the B-complex vitamins to give an overall feeling of well-being. It aids in the formation of mother's milk and is a key element in the production of enzymes needed to oxidize fats and to metabolize purines, including the antioxidant enzyme superoxide dismutase (SOD).

A deficiency of manganese (which is extremely rare) may lead to atherosclerosis, confusion, convulsions, eye problems, hearing problems, heart disorders, high cholesterol levels, hypertension, irritability, memory loss, muscle contractions, pancreatic damage, profuse perspiration, rapid pulse, tooth-grinding, tremors, and a tendency toward breast ailments.

SOURCES The largest quantities of manganese are found in avocados, nuts and seeds, seaweed, and whole grains. This mineral may also be found in blueberries, egg yolks, legumes, dried peas, pineapples, and green leafy vegetables. Herbs that contain manganese include alfalfa, burdock root, catnip, chamomile, chickweed, dandelion, eyebright, fennel seed, fenugreek, ginseng, hops, horsetail, lemongrass, mullein, parsley, peppermint, raspberry, red clover, rose hips, wild yam, yarrow, and yellow dock.

Molybdenum

This essential mineral is required in extremely small amounts for nitrogen metabolism. It aids in the final stages of the conversion of purines to uric acid. It promotes normal cell function, aids in the activation of certain enzymes, and is a component of the metabolic enzyme xanthine oxidase. Molybdenum is found in the liver, bones, and kidneys. It supports bone growth and strengthening of the teeth. A low intake is associated with mouth and gum disorders and cancer. A molybdenum deficiency may cause impotence in older men. People whose diets are high in refined and processed foods are at risk for deficiency.

SOURCES This trace mineral is found in beans, beef liver, cereal grains, dark green leafy vegetables, legumes, and peas.

COMMENTS Heat and moisture can change the action of supplemental molybdenum. A high intake of sulfur may decrease molybdenum levels. Excess amounts of molybdenum (over 15 milligrams daily) may interfere with copper metabolism.

CAUTIONS Do not take over 15 milligrams of molybdenum daily. Higher doses may lead to the development of gout.

Phosphorus

Phosphorus is needed for blood clotting, bone and tooth formation, cell growth, contraction of the heart muscle, normal heart rhythm, and kidney function. It also assists the body in the utilization of vitamins and the conversion of food to energy. A proper balance of magnesium, calcium, and phosphorus should be maintained at all times. If one of these minerals is present in either excessive or insufficient amounts, this will have adverse effects on the body.

Deficiencies of phosphorus are rare, but can lead to such symptoms as anxiety, bone pain, fatigue, irregular breathing, irritability, numbness, skin sensitivity, trembling, weakness, and weight changes.

SOURCES Phosphorus deficiency is rare because this mineral is found in most foods, especially processed cooked foods and carbonated soft drinks. Significant amounts of phosphorus are contained in asparagus; bran; brewer's yeast; corn; dairy products; eggs; fish; dried fruit; garlic; legumes; nuts; sesame, sunflower, and pumpkin seeds; meats; poultry; salmon; and whole grains.

COMMENTS Excessive amounts of phosphorus interfere with calcium uptake. A diet high in processed cooked foods and junk food is a common culprit. Vitamin D increases the effectiveness of phosphorus.

Potassium

This mineral is important for a healthy nervous system and a regular heart rhythm. It helps prevent stroke, aids in proper muscle contraction, and works with sodium to control the body's water balance. Potassium is important for chemical reactions within the cells and aids in maintaining stable blood pressure and in transmitting electrochemical impulses. A 1997 review of earlier studies showed that low potassium intake may be a significant factor in the development of high blood pressure. Potassium also regulates the transfer of nutrients through cell membranes. This function of potassium has been shown to decrease with age, which may account for some of the circulatory damage, lethargy, and weakness experienced by older people. Together with magnesium, potassium can help prevent calcium-oxalate kidney stones.

Signs of potassium deficiency include abnormally dry skin, acne, chills, cognitive impairment, constipation, depression, diarrhea, diminished reflex function, edema, nervousness, insatiable thirst, fluctuations in heartbeat, glucose intolerance, growth impairment, high cholesterol levels, insomnia, low blood pressure, muscular fatigue and weakness, nausea and vomiting, periodic headaches, proteinuria (protein in the urine), respiratory distress, and salt retention.

SOURCES Food sources of potassium include dairy foods, fish, fruit, legumes, meat, poultry, vegetables, and whole grains. High amounts are found in apricots, avocados, bananas, lima beans, blackstrap molasses, brewer's yeast, brown rice, dates, dulse, figs, dried fruit, garlic, nuts, potatoes, raisins, spinach, winter squash, torula yeast, wheat bran, yams, and yogurt. Herbs that contain potassium include catnip, hops, horsetail, nettle, plantain, red clover, sage, and skullcap.

COMMENTS Kidney disorders, diarrhea, and the use of diuretics or laxatives all disrupt potassium levels. Tobacco and caffeine reduce potassium absorption. Using large amounts of licorice over long periods can deplete the body's potassium supply.

Potassium is needed for hormone secretion. The secretion of stress hormones causes a decrease in the potassium-to-sodium ratio both inside and outside the cells. As a result, stress increases the body's potassium requirements.

Selenium

Selenium's principal function is to inhibit the oxidation of lipids (fats) as a component of the enzyme glutathione peroxidase. It is a vital antioxidant, especially when combined with vitamin E. It protects the immune system by preventing the formation of free radicals that can damage the body. (*See* chapter six—ANTIOXI-DANTS.) Selenium plays a vital role in regulating the effects of thyroid hormone on fat metabolism. It has also been found to function as a preventive against the formation of certain types of tumors. One study found that men who took 200 micrograms of selenium daily over a ten-year period had roughly half the risk of developing lung, prostate, and colorectal cancer as compared with men who did not.

Selenium and vitamin E act synergistically to aid in the production of antibodies and to help maintain a healthy heart and liver. This trace element is needed for pancreatic function and tissue elasticity. When combined with vitamin E and zinc, it may also provide relief from an enlarged prostate. Selenium supplementation has been found to protect the liver in people with alcoholic cirrhosis. Studies conducted at the University of Miami indicate that taking supplemental selenium may enhance the survival of people with AIDS by increasing both red and white blood cell counts. It has shown promise in the treatment of arthritis, cardiovascular disease, male infertility, cataracts, AIDS, and high blood pressure.

Selenium deficiency has been linked to cancer and heart disease. It has also been associated with exhaustion, growth impairment, high cholesterol levels, infections, liver impairment, pancreatic insufficiency, and sterility. Symptoms of excessively high selenium levels can include arthritis, brittle nails, garlicky breath odor, gastrointestinal disorders, hair loss, irritability, liver and kidney impairment, a metallic taste in the mouth, pallor, skin eruptions, tooth loss, and yellowish skin. Unless your health care provider prescribes it, do not take more than 400 micrograms daily.

SOURCES Selenium can be found in meat and grains, depending on the selenium content of the soil where the food is grown. Because New Zealand soils are low in selenium, cattle and sheep raised there have suffered a breakdown of muscle tissue, including the heart muscle. However, human intake of selenium there is adequate because of imported Australian wheat. The soil of much American farm land is low in selenium, resulting in selenium-deficient produce.

Selenium can be found in Brazil nuts, brewer's yeast, broccoli, brown rice, chicken, dairy products, dulse, garlic, kelp, liver, molasses, onions, salmon, seafood, torula yeast, tuna, vegetables, wheat germ, and whole grains. Herbs that contain selenium include alfalfa, burdock root, catnip, cayenne, chamomile, chickweed, fennel seed, fenugreek, garlic, ginseng, hawthorn berry, hops, horsetail, lemongrass, milk thistle, nettle, oat straw, parsley, peppermint, raspberry leaf, rose hips, sarsaparilla, uva ursi, yarrow, and yellow dock.

COMMENTS Taking up to 200 micrograms of selenium per day is considered safe for most people. However, you should *not* take more than 40 micrograms of supplemental selenium daily if you are pregnant.

Silicon

Silicon is the second most abundant element on the planet (oxygen is the first). It is necessary for the formation of collagen for bones and connective tissue; for healthy nails, skin, and hair; and for calcium absorption in the early stages of bone formation. It is needed to maintain flexible arteries, and plays a major role in preventing cardiovascular disease. Silicon counteracts the effects of aluminum on the body and is important in the prevention of Alzheimer's disease and osteoporosis. It stimulates the immune system and inhibits the aging process in tissues. Silicon levels decrease with aging, so elderly people need larger amounts.

SOURCES Foods that contain silicon include alfalfa, beets, brown rice, the herb horsetail, bell peppers, soybeans, leafy green vegetables, and whole grains.

COMMENTS Silicon is most commonly found in the form of silica, a compound of silicon and oxygen also known as silicon dioxide (SiO_2). Two good sources of silicon are Body Essential Silica Gel from Anton Huebner GmbH and BioSil from Jarrow Formulas.

Boron, calcium, magnesium, manganese, and potassium aid in the efficient utilization of silicon.

Sodium

Sodium is necessary for maintaining proper water balance and blood pH. It is also needed for stomach, nerve, and muscle function. Although sodium deficiency is rare—most people have adequate (if not excessive) levels of sodium in their bodies—it can occur. This condition is most likely to affect people who take diuretics for high blood pressure, especially if they simultaneously adhere to low-sodium diets. Some experts estimate that as many as 20 percent of elderly people who take diuretics may be deficient in sodium. In some cases of disorders such as fibromyalgia, studies have shown that moderate amounts of sodium may be needed as well (natural sea salt is recommended). Symptoms of sodium deficiency can include abdominal cramps, anorexia, confusion, dehydration, depression, dizziness, fatigue, flatulence, hallucinations, headache, heart palpitations, an impaired sense of taste, lethargy, low blood pressure, memory impairment, muscular weakness, nausea and vomiting, poor coordination, recurrent infections, seizures, and weight loss. Excessive sodium intake can result in edema, high blood pressure, potassium deficiency, and liver and kidney disease.

73

SOURCES Virtually all foods contain some sodium.

COMMENTS A proper balance of potassium and sodium is necessary for good health. Since most people consume too much sodium, they typically need more potassium as well. An imbalance between sodium and potassium can lead to heart disease.

Sulfur

An acid-forming mineral that is part of the chemical structure of the amino acids methionine, cysteine, taurine, and glutathione, sulfur disinfects the blood, helps the body to resist bacteria, and protects the protoplasm of cells. It aids in necessary oxidation reactions in the body, stimulates bile secretion, and protects against toxic substances. Because of its ability to protect against the harmful effects of radiation and pollution, sulfur slows the aging process. It is found in all body tissues, and is needed for the synthesis of collagen, a principal protein that gives the skin its structural integrity.

SOURCES Brussels sprouts, dried beans, cabbage, eggs, fish, garlic, kale, meats, onions, soybeans, turnips, and wheat germ contain sulfur, as do the herb horsetail and the amino acids cysteine, cystine, lysine, and methionine. Sulfur is also available in tablet and powder forms. Methylsufonylmethane (MSM) is a good form of sulfur.

COMMENTS Moisture and heat may destroy or change the action of sulfur in the body. Sulfur is one of the key substances that makes garlic the "king of herbs."

Vanadium

Vanadium is needed for cellular metabolism and for the formation of bones and teeth. It plays a role in growth and reproduction, and inhibits cholesterol synthesis. Vanadium has been shown to have the ability to improve insulin utilization, resulting in improved glucose tolerance. A vanadium deficiency may be linked to cardiovascular and kidney disease, impaired reproductive ability, and increased infant mortality. Vanadium is not easily absorbed. Athletes may require more of this trace mineral than nonathletes.

SOURCES Vanadium is found in dill, fish, olives, meat, radishes, snap beans, vegetable oils, and whole grains.

COMMENTS There may be an interaction between vanadium and chromium. If you take supplemental chromium and vanadium, take them at different times. Tobacco use decreases the uptake of vanadium.

Zinc

This essential mineral is important in prostate gland function and the growth of the reproductive organs. Zinc may help prevent acne and regulate the activity of oil glands. It is required for protein synthesis and collagen formation, and promotes a healthy immune system and the healing of wounds. Zinc also allows acuity of taste and smell. It protects the liver from chemical damage and is vital for bone formation. It is a constituent of insulin and many vital enzymes, including the antioxidant enzyme superoxide dismutase (SOD). It also helps to fight and prevent the formation of free radicals in other ways. A form of zinc called zinc monomethionine (zinc bound with the amino acid methionine), sold under the trademark OptiZinc, has been found to have antioxidant activity comparable to that of vitamin C, vitamin E, and beta-carotene. Zinc lozenges have been reported to be effective in relieving symptoms of the common cold and reducing the duration of colds.

Sufficient intake and absorption of zinc are needed to maintain the proper concentration of vitamin E in the blood. In addition, zinc increases the absorption of vitamin A. For optimum health, a proper 1-to-10 balance between copper and zinc levels should be maintained.

A deficiency of zinc may result in the loss of the senses of taste and smell. It can also cause fingernails to become thin, peel, and develop white spots. Other possible signs of zinc deficiency include acne, delayed sexual maturation, fatigue, growth impairment, hair loss, high cholesterol levels, impaired night vision, impotence, increased susceptibility to infection, infertility, memory impairment, a propensity to diabetes, prostate trouble, recurrent colds and flu, skin lesions, and slow wound healing.

SOURCES Zinc is found in the following food sources: brewer's yeast, dulse, egg yolks, fish, kelp, lamb, legumes, lima beans, liver, meats, mushrooms, oysters, pecans, poultry, pumpkin seeds, sardines, seafood, soy lecithin, soybeans, sunflower seeds, torula yeast, and whole grains. Herbs that contain zinc include alfalfa, burdock root, cayenne, chamomile, chickweed, dandelion, eyebright, fennel seed, hops, milk thistle, mullein, nettle, parsley, rose hips, sage, sarsaparilla, skullcap, and wild yam.

COMMENTS Zinc levels may be lowered by diarrhea, kidney disease, cirrhosis of the liver, diabetes, or the consumption of fiber, which causes zinc to be excreted through the intestinal tract. A significant amount of zinc is lost through perspiration. The consumption of hard water also can upset zinc levels. Compounds called phytates that are found in grains and legumes bind with zinc so that it cannot be absorbed. If you take both zinc and iron supplements, take them at different times. If these two minerals are taken together, they interfere with each other's activity.

CAUTIONS Do not take a total of more than 100 milligrams of zinc daily. While daily doses under 100 milligrams enhance the immune response, doses of more than 100 milligrams can depress the immune system.

Water

INTRODUCTION

Human beings can survive without food for thirty to forty days—about five weeks—but without water, life would end in three to five days. The average person's body is composed of approximately 70 percent water, although the water content varies considerably from person to person and even from one body part to another. The body's water supply is responsible for and involved in nearly every bodily process, including digestion, absorption, circulation, and excretion. Water is also the primary transporter of nutrients throughout the body and so is necessary for all building functions in the body. Water helps maintain normal body temperature and is essential for carrying waste material out of the body. Therefore, replacing the water that is continually being lost through sweating and elimination is very important.

A drop in the body's water content causes a decline in blood volume. The lowering of blood volume in turn triggers the hypothalamus, which is the brain's thirst center, to send out the demand for a drink. This causes a slight rise in the concentration of sodium in the blood. These changes quickly trigger a sensation of thirst. Unfortunately, people often consume only enough liquid to quench a dry or parched throat—not enough to cover all of their water loss. As a result, they can become dehydrated. As we age, the sense of thirst becomes dulled. At the same time, we have a lower percentage of reserve body water than we had when we were younger. This is why it is important to drink water even when you do not feel thirsty.

Quality water is beneficial for virtually all disorders known to humankind. Bowel and bladder problems, as well as headaches, can be reduced by drinking water. If not enough water is consumed, toxins can build up in the system, causing headaches. Water flushes these toxins out. Anxiety attacks, food intolerances, "acid stomach" and heartburn, muscle pains, colitis pain, hot flashes, and many other discomforts and disorders can be eased quickly by drinking a full glass of water. Chronic fatigue syndrome (CFS) is another disorder that necessitates consuming plenty of quality water daily to flush out toxins and other substances that contribute to muscle aches and extreme fatigue.

Without adequate water, we would poison ourselves with our own metabolic wastes. The kidneys remove waste products, such as uric acid, urea, and lactic acid, that must be dissolved in water. If there is not enough water available to remove these substances effectively, they may cause damage to the kidneys. Digestion and metabolism also rely on water for certain enzymatic and chemical reactions in the body. Water carries nutrients and oxygen to cells through the blood and is involved in the regulation of body temperature through perspiration. Water is especially important for people who have musculoskeletal problems such as arthritis, or who are athletic, as it lubricates the joints. Because lung tissue must be moist to facilitate oxygen intake and carbon dioxide excretion, water is essential for breathing. Approximately one pint of liquid is lost each day through exhaling. If you do not take in enough water to maintain fluid balance, every bodily function can be impaired. And the more active you are, the more water you must consume in order to keep your body's water level in balance.

Inadequate water consumption may contribute to excess body fat; poor muscle tone; digestive problems; poor functioning of many organs, including the brain; joint and muscle soreness; and, paradoxically, water retention. Consuming plenty of quality water can slow the aging process, and can prevent or improve arthritis, kidney stones, constipation, arteriosclerosis, obesity, glaucoma, cataracts, diabetes, hypoglycemia, and many other diseases. It is not expensive, and you should feel a difference quickly, but you must drink eight to ten full glasses of quality water daily.

Obtaining quality water would seem to be an easy matter. However, due to the numerous types of classifications water is given, the average consumer can easily be confused about what is available. This section offers a guide to understanding what the most commonly used classifications of water mean and how these different kinds of water may help or harm the body.

TAP WATER

Water that comes out of household taps or faucets is generally obtained either from surface water—water that has run off from ponds, creeks, streams, rivers, and lakes, and is collected in reservoirs—or from ground water—water that has filtered through the ground to the water table and is extracted by means of a well. Approximately half of the tap water in the United States comes from lakes, rivers, or other surface sources. Underground aquifers and municipal wells provide 35 percent of tap water, and the remaining 15 percent comes from private wells.

The Safety of Tap Water

Most people assume that when they turn on the kitchen tap, they are getting clean, safe, healthy drinking water. Unfortunately, this often is not the case. Regardless of the original source of tap water, it is vulnerable to a number of different types of impurities, and may be full of harmful chemicals and inorganic minerals that the body cannot use. Some undesirable substances found in water, including radon, fluoride, and arsenic, as well as iron, lead, copper, and other heavy metals, can occur naturally. Other contaminants, such as fertilizers, asbestos, cyanides, herbicides, pesticides, and industrial chemicals, may leach into ground water through the soil, or into any tap water from plumbing pipes. Many of these chemicals have been linked to cancer and other disorders. Water can also contain biological contaminants, including viruses, bacteria, and parasites. Still other substances, including chlorine, carbon, lime, phosphates, soda ash, and aluminum sulfate, are intentionally added to public water supplies to kill bacteria, adjust pH, and eliminate cloudiness, among other things.

A study conducted by the Natural Resources Defense Council found that 18,500 of the nation's water systems (serving some 45 million Americans) violated safe drinking water laws at some point during 1994 or 1995. The council's report blamed contaminated water for some 900,000 illnesses a year, including 100 deaths. Even if the levels of individual substances in water are well within "allowable" limits, the total of all contaminants present may still be harmful to your health. And private wells may not be regulated at all, except at the local level.

The greatest concerns about water quality today focus on chlorine, pesticides, and parasites. Chlorine has long been added to public water supplies to kill disease-causing bacteria. However, the levels of chlorine in drinking water today can be quite high, and some byproducts of chlorine are known carcinogens. As a result, the U.S. Environmental Protection Agency (EPA) is considering steps to reduce the level of chlorine in drinking water, but is facing opposition from industry groups.

Pesticides pose a risk in any area where the tap water is extracted from an underground source. These chemicals are suspected of causing, or at least contributing to, an increased incidence of cancer, especially breast cancer. Some scientists believe this may be because certain pesticides can mimic the action of the sex hormone estrogen in the body. Others point to the fact that toxins in the body tend to accumulate in fatty tissues, and the human breast is composed largely of fatty tissue. The pesticide problem is a particular concern in areas where agriculture is (or was) a major part of the economy. These chemicals are persistent. Residues from pesticides used decades ago may still be present in water coming out of the tap today, and may pose a risk to health.

Long considered a problem limited to poor, developing countries, the presence of bacteria and parasites in drinking water—especially a parasite called *cryptosporidium*—is becoming a serious problem in the United States today. In April 1993, as many as 370,000 people in and around Milwaukee, Wisconsin, were stricken by the parasite *Cryptosporidium parvum* from the city's water supply. Thousands suffered from severe diarrhea, and up to 100 deaths were attributed to the outbreak. These "unacceptable" levels of cryptosporidia, most likely from agricultural runoff, forced users of the public water system to boil their tap water before using it. The same organism has created controversy over the safety of the water in New York City; many people with weakened immune systems have charged that cryptosporidia in the city's water have made them sick, even though local officials insist that the water is safe to drink. For people with HIV or AIDS, cryptosporidia can be lethal. The chlorine added to water to kill bacteria is not effective at killing these parasites. In addition to cryptosporidiosis, giardiasis, also caused by an intestinal parasite, can be contracted through drinking water and is an increasing problem. Like cryptosporidia, giardia resist the effects of chlorine (outbreaks have occurred in areas where the water is routinely chlorine-treated) and pose a more serious problem for people with diminished immune response. Indeed, because of increasing concern over the danger contaminated drinking water poses for people with compromised immune systems, the U.S. Centers for Disease Control and Prevention (CDC) and the EPA have issued suggestions that immunocompromised individuals boil tap water for at least one minute before use, use an appropriate filtration system, or buy quality bottled drinking water.

More than one-third of all community water systems have been cited for failure to meet the EPA's water safety standards or treatment technique, monitoring, or reporting requirements. Consumer activist Ralph Nader's Center for Study of Responsive Law issued a study in 1988 entitled *Troubled Waters On Tap: Organic Chemicals in Public Drinking Water Systems and the Failure or Regulation* that identified over 2,100 contaminants in tap water in the United States. And according to a study released in 1995, 54 million Americans drank tap water that was contaminated by feces, radiation, lead, or dangerous parasites at some time between 1993 and 1994.

If you receive your water from a municipal water source, that utility is now required to send an assessment of the water, including information about where it comes from, any contaminants that have been found in it, and any health risk associated with substances in the water. This should be sent to you in your water bill on an annual basis. Whatever the source of your water, it is important to know some warning signs of bad water. Watch for cloudiness or murkiness in water. Chlorination can cause some cloudiness, but it usually clears if the water is left to stand, whereas bacterial or sedimentary cloudiness will remain. Foaming may be caused by bacterial contamination, by floating particles of sediment, or by soaps or detergents. Bacteria can be destroyed by boiling water for at least five minutes, while sediment should settle out if you let the water stand for several hours. Strange smells or tastes in water that was previously fine could mean chemical contamination. However, many toxic hazards that work their way into water do not change its taste, smell, or appearance.

Hard Versus Soft Water

Hard water, found in various parts of the country, contains relatively high concentrations of the minerals calcium and magnesium. The presence of these minerals prevents soap from lathering and results in filmy sediment being deposited on hair, clothing, pipes, dishes, washtubs, and anything else that comes into regular contact with the water. It also affects the taste. Hard water can be annoying, and though some studies have shown that deaths from heart disease may be lower in areas where the drinking water is hard, we believe that the calcium found in hard water is not good for the heart, arteries, or bones. Hard water deposits its calcium and other minerals on the *outside* of these structures, while it is the calcium and magnesium found *within* these structures that are beneficial to the body.

Soft water can be naturally soft or it may be hard water that has been treated to remove the calcium and magnesium. Standard water-softening systems work by using pressure to pass the water through exchange media to exchange "hard" calcium and magnesium ions for "soft" sodium or potassium ions. Most use either sodium chloride or potassium chloride for this purpose. The pri-

MTBE AND DRINKING WATER

Since 1979, methyl tertiary butyl ether (MTBE) has been added to gasoline to increase its oxygen content. It took the place of lead as an octane enhancer, and was supposed to reduce the problems of both smog and carbon monoxide in the atmosphere. The Clean Air Act of 1990 required the use of reformulated gasoline, or RFG, in certain parts of the country, with the goal of reducing air pollution in those areas. RFG accounts for some 30 percent of gasoline sold in the United States, and MTBE is now added to over 80 percent of RFG fuel.

According to a disturbing report aired on the CBS television program *60 Minutes* on January 16, 2000, this measure to improve air quality has, ironically, given Americans yet another reason to be concerned about the safety of their drinking water supply. MTBE has been seeping into all our water supplies, both surface and underground, at an alarming rate. It has been found in storm water in 592 samples collected in sixteen cities between 1991 and 1995. The primary sources of the MTBE that ends up in water systems are leaking gasoline tanks and reservoirs, drinking water lakes, and rivers where gasoline-powered recreational watercraft are permitted. Less than one-tenth of a gallon (roughly 12 ounces) of MTBE is capable of contaminat-

continued on next page

mary benefit of softening is in improved cleaning properties for the water and less mineral buildup inside household pipes and equipment. One potentially serious problem with artificially softened water is that it is more likely than hard water to dissolve the lining of pipes. This poses an especially significant threat if pipes are made of lead. Another threat comes from certain plastic and galvanized pipes, which contain cadmium, a toxic heavy metal. These types of pipes are rarely used in construction today, but they may be present in older buildings that have not undergone extensive renovation. But leaching from pipes can be a problem with today's copper pipes as well. Dangerous levels of copper, iron, zinc, and arsenic can leach into softened water from copper pipes. Another potential problem with artificially softened water is of concern to

continued from previous page
ing 13 million gallons of drinking water. It is estimated that over 1 million gallons of fuel are deposited, unburned, into the water supply each year as a result of recreational boating.

Few long-term studies have been done on this chemical, but what little research there is indicates that MTBE is a likely human carcinogen and immune-system depressant. Certainly, tests on rats have provided evidence that MTBE is a cancer-causing agent. To date, drinking water supplies in the states of California, New York, Maine, Pennsylvania, Connecticut, and Rhode Island have been closed down due to contamination by MTBE (boiling drinking water does not help purge it of this agent). MTBE-contaminated tap water can cause problems even if you do not drink it. This chemical can also be absorbed through the skin when showering and can be inhaled as a vapor in the air. Possible effects of inhaling MTBE include headaches, burning of the nose and throat, dizziness, nausea, asthma, and respiratory problems. The possible effects on wildlife have not yet been documented.

Only recently has the Environmental Protection Agency (EPA) considered making it mandatory to test for MTBE in drinking water, but the likelihood is that it will not be until the year 2010 that the EPA will make a determination on the continued use of MTBE.

people with kidney failure. People with kidney failure must restrict their intake of potassium. Potassium-based water-softening systems can therefore pose a danger to such individuals.

Fluoridation

For many years now, controversy has raged over whether fluoride should be added to drinking water. As early as 1961, as recorded in the Congressional Record, fluoride was exposed as a lethal poison in our nation's water supply. Proponents say that fluoride occurs naturally and helps develop and maintain strong bones and teeth. Opponents to fluoridation contend that when fluoridated water is consumed regularly, toxic levels of fluorine, the poisonous substance from which fluoride is derived, build up in the body, causing irreparable harm to the immune system. The Delaney Congressional Investigation Committee, the government body charged with monitoring additives and other substances in the food supply, has stated that "fluoridation is mass medication without parallel in the history of medicine."

Meanwhile, no convincing scientific proof has ever been generated that fluoridated water makes for stronger bones and teeth. It is known, however, that chronic fluoride use results in numerous health problems, including osteoporosis and osteomalacia, and also damages teeth and leaves them mottled. The salts used to fluoridate our nation's water supply, sodium fluoride and fluorosalicic acid, are industrial byproducts that are never found in nature. They are also notoriously toxic compounds, so much so that they are used in rat poison and insecticides. The naturally occurring form of fluoride, calcium fluoride, is not toxic—but this form of fluoride is not used to fluoridate water.

Today, more than half the cities in the United States fluoridate their water supplies. In many states, it is required. Although many ailments and disorders—including Down syndrome, mottled teeth, and cancer—have been linked to fluoridated water, fluoridation has become the standard rather than the exception.

The fluoride added to tap water can be a problem. Individuals have different levels of tolerance for toxins such as fluoride. In addition, many water sources have levels of fluoride higher than one part per million, the level generally recognized as safe and originally set as the acceptable limit by the EPA. After the EPA learned that water in many towns had natural fluoride levels much higher than this, the permissible fluoride limit was raised—quadrupled, in fact—to four parts per million. And this is in addition to fluoride encountered from other sources. Fluoride is the thirteenth most widely distributed element on earth, so it can turn up just about anywhere—in vegetables and meats, for example. Since so many local water supplies are fluoridated, there is a good chance that virtually any packaged food product made with water, such as soft drinks and reconstituted juices, contains fluoride. Additional fluorides are widely used in toothpaste products, so it is easy to see how many Americans may be ingesting excessive amounts of this potentially toxic substance.

If your tap water contains fluoride, and you wish to remove it, you can use a reverse osmosis, distillation, or activated alumina filtration system to eliminate almost all of the fluoride from your water.

Water Analysis

Not all drinking water contains significant amounts of toxic substances. Some places rate higher in water safety than others. In addition, not all cities and towns process their water supplies the same way. Some do nothing at all to their water. Others add chemicals to the water to kill bacteria. Still others filter their water. It is up to the individual to find out how local drinking water is treated and to determine how safe the water coming out of the tap is.

The EPA has defined pure water as "bacteriologically safe" water, and it recommends—but does not require—that tap water have a pH between 6.5 and 8.5. This allows for a great deal of leeway in what passes as acceptable water. If you are concerned about the safety of the water coming out of your tap, you can contact your local water officials or local health department, which may test your tap water free of charge. In some cases, you may have to contact your state's water supply or health department. Typically, however, these agencies test the water only for bacteria levels, not for toxic substances. Therefore, you might want to contact a commercial laboratory or local state university laboratory to test your water for its chemical content. If you find that your tap water is unacceptable either because of its taste or because of its toxic chemical content, you may choose to use one of the alternative water supplies described in this section.

The Water Quality Association is prepared to answer questions about the various types of water and methods of water treatment. In addition, the EPA operates the toll-free Safe Drinking Water Hotline, which can help you to locate an office or laboratory in your area that does certified water testing. There are also a number of laboratories that will send a self-addressed container for you to fill and return by mail for testing. The cost starts at thirty-five to forty dollars per tap. Results are usually available in two to three weeks.

To help you understand the results of water testing, you should obtain information on the EPA's Recommended Maximum Contaminant Levels. This and other water-quality information is available from NSF International, Inc. (formerly the National Sanitation Foundation) and the Water Quality Association.

Improving Tap Water

Tap water can be improved in several ways. Heating tap water to a rolling boil and keeping it there for three to five minutes will kill bacteria and parasites. However, most people find boiling their drinking water too impractical and time-consuming. In addition, this procedure has the effect of concentrating whatever lead is present in the water, and the water must then be refrigerated if it is to be used for drinking. The taste of chlorinated tap water can be improved by keeping the water in an uncovered pitcher for several hours to allow the chlorine taste and odor to dissipate. Water can also be aerated in a blender to remove chlorine and other chemicals. Nevertheless, neither of these last two methods will improve the quality of the water—only the taste.

Filtration is a means by which contaminants in water are removed, rendering the water cleaner and better tasting. There are many different ways in which water can be filtered. Nature filters water as the water runs through streams and as it seeps down through the soil and rocks to the water table. As water passes through the earth or over the rocks in a stream, the bacteria in the water leech into the rocks and are replaced with minerals such as calcium and magnesium.

There are also man-made ways of filtering water. There are three basic types of filters available: absorbent types, which use materials such as carbon to pick up impurities; microfiltration systems, which run water through filters with tiny pores to catch and eliminate contaminants (the filter may be made of any of a number of different materials); and special media such as ion-exchange resins that are designed to remove heavy metals. Filters are often arranged in series, so that the filtering media that are most effective for specific types of contaminants can be used. The primary advantage of filters is relatively low cost and ease of use.

Water filtration systems vary in effectiveness. Two types that are considered good are reverse osmosis and ceramic filtration systems. In reverse osmosis filtering, the water is forced through a semipermeable membrane, while charged particles and larger molecules are repelled. It is the best system for treating water that is brackish (high in salt), high in nitrates, and loaded with inorganic heavy metals such as iron and lead. However, no filter can remove absolutely all contaminants. Each pore of even the finest filter is large enough for some viruses to permeate. To remove parasites such as cryptosporidia, the EPA and CDC recommend purchasing a filter that has an NSF rating for parasite reduction *and* that has an absolute pore size of one micron or smaller.

Other water treatment systems that remove various contaminants include distillers and ultraviolet treatment units. The latter are used to kill bacteria and viruses in water. Each treatment method has its advantages and disadvantages (*see* Home Water Treatment Methods, below), but using a combination of methods can result in the best overall quality drinking water. Even the quality and taste of distilled water can be improved by passing the water through a charcoal/carbon filter as a final step.

Before you purchase a water treatment unit, contact NSF International or the Water Quality Association. These nonprofit testing and certification organizations verify manufacturers' claims and certify that the materials used are nontoxic and structurally sound. They conduct periodic unannounced audits of the products they certify to ensure that the products still comply with standards.

One manufacturer of home distillation units that has certification for different models from both NSF International and the Water Quality Association is Waterwise, Inc. This company offers options combining both pre-distillation and post-distillation carbon filtration, and also manufactures a showerhead water filtration system that rids shower water of chlorine and various other contaminants. Pure Water, Inc. manufactures home and small business distillation systems that are in use throughout the world. Reverse osmosis system manufacturers whose products can claim certification by NSF International and the Water Quality Association include EcoWater Systems and Rainsoft.

HOME WATER TREATMENT METHODS

Activated carbon

COST Faucet-mounted or pour-through unit: $20–$60
Countertop unit: $89–200
Under-sink unit: $75–$600
Whole-house system: $499–$1,250

HOW IT WORKS Water is filtered through a carbon trap that absorbs the contaminants.

WHAT IT DOES Reduces levels of chlorine, herbicides, lead, hydrogen sulfide, and volatile organic chemicals (VOCs). Also reduces color and turbidity.

Carbon filtration

COST Faucet-mounted unit: $25
Under-counter unit: $300 and up

HOW IT WORKS Passes water through a charcoal or solid carbon block and captures contaminants. When carbon sites fill up, the filter cartridge is replaced.

WHAT IT DOES Reduces levels of chlorine, organic chemicals, and pesticides. Also reduces bad taste and odors.

continued on next page

89

BOTTLED WATER

Because of concerns over the safety and health effects of tap water, many people today are turning to bottled water. Bottled water is usually classified by its source (spring, spa, geyser, public water supply, etc.), by its mineral content (containing at least 250 parts per million of dissolved solids), and/or by the type of treatment it has undergone (deionized, steam-distilled, etc.). Because there is a lot of overlapping among these criteria, some water fits more than one classification. In addition, most states have no rules governing appropriate labeling, so some bottled water claims may be misleading or incorrect.

While the EPA is charged with the regulation of public water supplies, it is the U.S. Food and Drug Administration (FDA) that

continued from previous page

Distillation

COST Countertop unit: $99–$995
Free-standing unit: $599–$1,020
Whole-house system: $799–$4,500

HOW IT WORKS Raises water temperature to boiling, leaving contaminants behind. Purified water vapor condenses to liquid.

WHAT IT DOES Reduces levels of arsenic, cadmium, chromium, iron, lead, giardia cysts, nitrate, and sulfate. Also reduces turbidity.

Reverse osmosis

COST Countertop unit: $150–$250
Under-sink unit: $530–$1,500

HOW IT WORKS Forces pressurized water through a contamination-rejecting membrane; sends improved water to holding tank.

WHAT IT DOES Reduces levels of arsenic, cadmium, iron, chlorine, color, lead, giardia, giardia cysts, nitrate, radium, and sulfate. Also reduces color and turbidity.

Water softener

COST Whole-house system: $950–$3,500

HOW IT WORKS Replaces calcium and magnesium with sodium to "soften" the water.

WHAT IT DOES Reduces levels of calcium, iron, and radium.

has responsibility for overseeing the quality and safety of bottled drinking water. The FDA defines the terms used to describe bottled drinking waters in specific requirements last revised in April 1997, making the choices for the consumer somewhat clearer than in the past. The FDA regulations for bottled water allow for the various terms that have been defined to be used with one another if bottled water meets more than one definition, so it is possible for some water labels to include a number of different terms.

All the terms that are legally necessary to describe bottled drinking water are discussed in the paragraphs that follow. Any term you find on a label that is *not* defined or included here is a marketing slogan added to entice the consumer to buy the product. It can mean anything that the manufacturer of the product says it means.

Artesian Water

Artesian water, or artesian well water, is water drawn from a well where the water is brought to the surface by natural pressure or flow.

Bottled Water

Bottled water, or bottled drinking water, is water that is intended for human consumption and that is sealed in bottles or other containers with no added ingredients except for optional antimicrobial agents. These must be identified on the label. If bottled water comes from a community water system or from a municipal source, this information must appear on the label. About 25 percent of bottled waters now sold come from the same water supplies that flow into some areas' household taps.

Deionized or Demineralized Water

When the electric charge of a molecule of water has been neutralized by the addition or removal of electrons, the resulting water is called *deionized* or *demineralized*. The deionization process removes nitrates and the minerals calcium and magnesium, in addition to the heavy metals cadmium, barium, lead, mercury, and some forms of radium.

Ground Water

This is water that comes from underground, in the water table, that is under pressure equal to or greater than atmospheric pressure, and that does not come into contact with surface water. Ground water must be pumped mechanically for bottling.

Mineral Water

Mineral water is water containing not less than 250 parts per million total dissolved solids (TDS), originating from a geologically and physically protected underground water source or spring that has been tapped at the spring opening or through a borehole. Mineral water is distinguished from other types of water by constant levels and relative proportions of minerals and trace elements at its source, allowing for seasonal variations. No minerals may be added to this water. If the TDS content of mineral water is below 500 parts per million, the water may be labeled *low mineral content*. If it is greater than 1,500 parts per million, the label *high mineral content* may be used.

Depending on where the source is, the minerals the water contains will vary. If you are suffering from a deficiency of certain minerals and are drinking mineral water for therapeutic reasons, you must be aware of which minerals are in the particular brand of water you drink. If you are drinking mineral water containing minerals that you do not lack, you could be doing yourself more harm than good.

Most mineral waters are carbonated. However, some sparkling waters, such as club soda, are called mineral waters because the manufacturer added bicarbonates, citrates, and sodium phosphates to filtered or distilled tap water.

Natural Spring Water

The term *natural spring water* on a bottled water label doesn't tell you where the water came from, only that the mineral content of the water has not been altered. It may or may not have been filtered or otherwise treated. While the number of gallons of "natural spring water" flowing through water coolers and from bottles has more than doubled in recent years, the meaning of these words on a label has been firmly defined only since the final changes in the FDA bottled drinking water regulations have been in place.

Spring water is water that comes from an underground formation from which water flows naturally to the surface of the earth. It must be collected at the spring or through a borehole tapping the underground formation that feeds the spring. To meet the definition of *spring,* there must be natural force bringing the water to the surface opening. The location of the spring must be identified on the label of any water labeled as spring water.

If you use a water cooler for bottled spring water, you should be sure to clean the cooler once a month to destroy bacteria. Run a 50-50 mixture of hydrogen peroxide and baking soda through the reservoir and spigots, then remove the residue by rinsing the cooler with four or more gallons of tap water.

Sparkling Water

This is bottled water that contains the same amount of carbon dioxide that it had at emergence from the water source. It can be a healthful alternative to soda and alcoholic beverages, but if it is loaded with fructose and other sweeteners, it may be no better than soda pop. Read labels before you buy. Soda water, seltzer water, and tonic water are *not* considered bottled waters. They are regulated separately, may contain sugar and calories, and are considered soft drinks.

Understanding where the carbonation in sparkling water comes from isn't always easy. A "naturally sparkling water" must get its carbonation from the same source as the water. If a water is "carbonated natural water," that means the carbonation came from a source other than the one that supplied the water. That doesn't mean the water is of poor quality. It can still be called "natural" because its mineral content is the same as when it came from the ground, even though it has been carbonated from a separate source. People suffering from intestinal disorders or ulcers should avoid drinking carbonated water because it may be irritating to the gastrointestinal tract.

Steam-Distilled Water

Distillation involves vaporizing water by boiling it. The steam rises, leaving behind most of the bacteria, viruses, chemicals, minerals, and pollutants from the water. The steam is then moved into a condensing chamber, where it is cooled and condensed to become distilled water.

Once consumed, steam-distilled water leaches inorganic minerals rejected by the cells and tissues out of the body.

We believe that only steam-distilled or reverse osmosis-filtered water should be consumed. They should be used not only for drinking, but in cooking as well, because foods such as pasta, rice, and beans can absorb chemicals found in unpurified water.

Flavor can be added to distilled water by adding 1 to 2 tablespoons of raw apple cider vinegar (obtained from a health food store) per gallon of distilled water. Vinegar is an excellent solvent and aids in digestion. Lemon juice is another good flavoring agent, and has cleansing properties as well. For added minerals, you can add mineral drops to steam-distilled water. Concentrace from Trace Minerals Research is a good product for this purpose. Add 1 ¼ teaspoons of mineral drops to every 5 gallons of water.

FIVE

Amino Acids

INTRODUCTION

Amino acids are the chemical units or "building blocks," as they are popularly called, that make up proteins. They also are the end products of protein digestion, or *hydrolysis*. Amino acids contain about 16 percent nitrogen. Chemically, this is what distinguishes them from the other two basic nutrients, sugars and fatty acids, which do not contain nitrogen.

To understand how vital amino acids are, you must understand how essential proteins are to life. It is protein that provides the structure for all living things. Every living organism, from the largest animal to the tiniest microbe, is composed of protein. And in its various forms, protein participates in the vital chemical processes that sustain life.

Proteins are a necessary part of every living cell in the body. Next to water, protein makes up the greatest portion of our body weight. In the human body, protein substances make up the muscles, ligaments, tendons, organs, glands, nails, hair, and many vital body fluids, and are essential for the growth of bones. The enzymes and hormones that catalyze and regulate all bodily processes are proteins. Proteins help to regulate the body's water balance and maintain the proper internal pH. They assist in the exchange of nutrients between the intercellular fluids and the tissues, blood, and lymph. A deficiency of protein can upset the body's fluid balance, causing edema. Proteins form the structural basis of chromosomes, through which genetic information is passed from parents to off-spring. The genetic "code" contained in each cell's DNA is actually information for how to make that cell's proteins.

Proteins are chains of amino acids linked together by what are called *peptide bonds*. Each individual type of protein is composed of a specific group of amino acids in a specific chemical arrange-ment. It is the particular amino acids present and the way in which they are linked together in sequence that gives the proteins that make up the various tissues their unique functions and characters. Each protein in the body is tailored for a specific need; proteins are not interchangeable.

The proteins that make up the human body are not obtained directly from the diet. Rather, dietary protein is broken down into its constituent amino acids, which the body then uses to build the specific proteins it needs. Thus, it is the amino acids rather than protein that are the essential nutrients.

In addition to those that combine to form the body's proteins, there are other amino acids that are important in metabolic func-tions. Some, such as citrulline, glutathione, ornithine, and tau-rine, can be similar to (or byproducts of) the protein-building amino acids. Some act as neurotransmitters or as precursors of neurotransmitters, the chemicals that carry information from one nerve cell to another. Certain amino acids are thus necessary for the brain to receive and send messages. Unlike many other sub-stances, neurotransmitters are able to pass through the *blood-brain barrier*. This is a kind of defensive shield designed to protect the brain from toxins and foreign invaders that may be circulating in the bloodstream. The endothelial cells that make up the walls of the capillaries in the brain are much more tightly meshed together than are those of capillaries elsewhere in the body. This prevents many substances, especially water-based substances, from diffus-ing through the capillary walls into brain tissue. Because certain amino acids can pass through this barrier, they can be used by the brain to communicate with nerve cells elsewhere in the body.

Amino acids also enable vitamins and minerals to perform their jobs properly. Even if vitamins and minerals are absorbed and as-similated by the body, they cannot be effective unless the necessary amino acids are present. For example, low levels of the amino acid tyrosine may lead to iron deficiency. Deficiency and/or impaired metabolism of the amino acids methionine and taurine has been linked to allergies and autoimmune disorders. Many elderly people suffer from depression or neurological problems that may be associated with deficiencies of the amino acids tyrosine, tryptophan, phenylalanine, and histidine, and also of the *branched-chain amino acids*—valine, isoleucine, and leucine. These are amino acids that can be used to provide energy directly to muscle tissue. High doses of branched-chain amino acids have been used in hospitals to treat people suffering from trauma and infection. Some people are born with an inability to metabolize the branched-chain amino acids. This potentially life-threatening condition, branched-chain ketoaciduria (often referred to as *maple syrup urine disease* because keto acids released into the urine cause it to smell like maple syrup) can result in neurological damage and necessitates a special diet, including a synthetic infant formula that does not contain leucine, isoleucine, or valine.

There are approximately twenty-eight commonly known amino acids that are combined in various ways to create the hundreds of different types of proteins present in all living things. In the human body, the liver produces about 80 percent of the amino acids needed. The remaining 20 percent must be obtained from the diet. These are called the *essential amino acids*. The essential amino acids that must enter the body through diet are histidine, isoleucine, leucine, lysine, methionine, phenylalanine, threonine, tryptophan, and valine. The nonessential amino acids, which can be manufactured in the body from other amino acids obtained from dietary sources, include alanine, arginine, asparagine, aspartic acid, citrulline, cysteine, cystine, gamma-aminobutyric acid, glutamic acid, glutamine, glycine, ornithine, proline, serine, taurine, and tyrosine. The fact that they are termed "nonessential" does not mean that they are not necessary, only that they need not be obtained through the diet because the body can manufacture them as needed. And nonessential amino acids can become "essential" under certain conditions. For instance, the nonessential amino acids cysteine and tyrosine are made from the essential amino acids methionine and phenylalanine. If methionine and phenylalanine are not available in sufficient quantities, cysteine and tyrosine then become essential in the diet.

The processes of assembling amino acids to make proteins, and of breaking down proteins into individual amino acids for the body's use, are continuous ones. When we need more enzyme proteins, the body produces more enzyme proteins; when we need more cells, the body produces more proteins for cells. These different types of proteins are produced as the need arises. Should the body become depleted of its reserves of any of the essential amino acids, it would not be able to produce the proteins that require those amino acids. An inadequate supply of even one essential amino acid can hinder the synthesis, and reduce body levels, of necessary proteins. This can result in negative nitrogen balance, an unhealthy condition in which the body excretes more nitrogen than it assimilates. Further, *all* of the essential amino acids must be present simultaneously in the diet in order for the other amino acids to be utilized—otherwise, the body remains in negative nitrogen balance. A lack of vital proteins in the body can cause problems ranging from indigestion to depression to stunted growth.

How could such a situation occur? More easily than you might think. Many factors can contribute to deficiencies of essential amino acids, even if you eat a well-balanced diet that contains enough protein. Impaired absorption, infection, trauma, stress, drug use, age, and imbalances of other nutrients can all affect the availability of essential amino acids in the body. Insufficient intake of vitamins and minerals, especially vitamin C, can interfere with the absorption of amino acids in the lower part of the small intestines. Vitamin B_6 is needed also, for the transport of amino acids in the body.

If your diet is *not* properly balanced—that is, if it fails to supply adequate amounts of the essential amino acids—sooner or later, this will become apparent as some type of physical disorder.

This does not mean, however, that eating a diet containing enormous amounts of protein is the answer. In fact, it is unhealthy. Excess protein puts undue stress on the kidneys and the liver, which are faced with processing the waste products of protein metabolism. Nearly half of the amino acids in dietary protein are transformed into glucose by the liver and utilized to provide needed energy to the cells. This process results in a waste product, ammonia. Ammonia is toxic to the body, so the body protects itself by having the liver turn the ammonia into a much less toxic compound, urea, which is then carried through the bloodstream, filtered out by the kidneys, and excreted.

As long as protein intake is not too great and the liver is working properly, ammonia is neutralized almost as soon as it is produced, so it does no harm. However, if there is too much ammonia for the liver to cope with—as a result of too much protein consumption, poor digestion, and/or a defect in liver function—toxic levels may accumulate. Strenuous exercise also tends to promote the accumulation of excess ammonia. This may put a person at risk for serious health problems, including encephalopathy (brain disease) or hepatic coma. Abnormally high levels of urea can also cause problems, including inflamed kidneys and back pain. Therefore, it is not the quantity but the quality of protein in the diet that is important (see chapter one—NUTRITION, DIET, AND WELLNESS).

It is possible to take supplements containing amino acids, both essential and nonessential. For certain disorders, taking supplements of specific amino acids can be very beneficial. When you take a specific amino acid or amino acid combination, it supports the metabolic pathway involved in your particular illness. Vegetarians, especially vegans, would be wise to take a formula containing all of the essential amino acids to ensure that their protein requirements are met.

WHAT'S ON THE SHELVES

Supplemental amino acids are available in combination with various multivitamin formulas, as protein mixtures, in a wide variety of food supplements, and in a number of amino acid formulas. They can be purchased as capsules, tablets, liquids, and powders. Most amino acid supplements are derived from animal protein, yeast protein, or vegetable protein. Crystalline free-form amino acids are generally extracted from a variety of grain products. Brown rice bran is a prime source, although cold-pressed yeast and milk proteins are also used.

Free-form means the amino acid is in its purest form. Free-form amino acids need no digestion and are absorbed directly into the bloodstream. These white crystalline amino acids are stable at room temperature and decompose when heated to temperatures of 350°F to 660°F (180°C to 350°C). They are rapidly absorbed and do not come from potentially allergenic food sources. For best results, choose encapsulated powders or powder.

When choosing amino acid supplements, look for products that contain USP (U.S. Pharmacopeia) pharmaceutical-grade L-crystalline amino acids. Most of the amino acids (except for glycine) can appear in two forms, the chemical structure of one being the mirror image of the other. These are called the D- and L- forms—for example, D-cystine and L-cystine. The "D" stands for *dextro* (Latin for "right") and the "L" for *levo* (Latin for "left"); these terms denote the direction of the rotation of the spiral that is the chemical structure of the molecule. Proteins in animal and plant tissue are made from the L-forms of amino acids (with the exception of phenylalanine, which is also used in the form of DL-phenylalanine, a mixture of the D- and L- forms). Thus, with respect to supplements of amino acids, products containing the L-forms of amino acids are considered to be more compatible with human biochemistry.

Each amino acid has specific functions in the body. The many functions and possible symptoms of deficiency of twenty-eight amino acids and related compounds are described below. When taking amino acids individually for healing purposes, take them on an empty stomach to avoid making them compete for absorption with the amino acids present in foods. When taking individual amino acids, it is best to take them in the morning or between meals, with small amounts of vitamin B_6 and vitamin C to enhance absorption. When taking an amino acid complex that includes all of the essential amino acids, it is best to take it one-half hour away from a meal, either before or after. If you are taking individual amino acids, it is wise also to take a full amino acid complex, including both essential and nonessential amino acids, at a different time. This is the best way to assure you have adequate amounts of all the necessary amino acids.

Be aware that individual amino acids should not be taken for long periods of time. A good rule to follow is to alternate the individual amino acids that fit your needs and back them up with an amino acid complex, taking the supplements for two months and then discontinuing them for two months. Moderation is the key. Some amino acids have potentially toxic effects when taken in high doses (over 6,000 milligrams per day) and may cause neurological damage. These include aspartic acid, glutamic acid, homocysteine, serine, and tryptophan. Cysteine can be toxic if taken in amounts over 1,000 milligrams per day. Do not give supplemental amino acids to a child, or take doses of any amino acid in excess of the amount recommended unless specifically directed to do so by your health care provider.

Some recommended amino acid products include the following:

- A/G-Pro from Miller Pharmacal Group, a complete amino acid and mineral supplement.
- Anabolic Amino Balance and Muscle Octane from Anabol Naturals. Anabolic Amino Balance is a complex of twenty-three free-form amino acids. Muscle Octane is a blend of free-form branched-chain amino acids (L-leucine, L-valine, and L-isoleucine). Anabol Naturals also produces free-form single amino acids.
- Amino Blend from Carlson Laboratories, a complex containing twenty amino acids, both essential and nonessential.

101

Alanine

Alanine plays a major role in the transfer of nitrogen from peripheral tissue to the liver. It aids in the metabolism of glucose, a simple carbohydrate that the body uses for energy. It also guards against the buildup of toxic substances that are released in the muscle cells when muscle protein is broken down to quickly meet energy needs, such as happens with aerobic exercise. Epstein-Barr virus and chronic fatigue have been associated with excessive alanine levels and low levels of tyrosine and phenylalanine. One form of alanine, beta-alanine, is a constituent of pantothenic acid (vitamin B_5) and coenzyme A, a vital catalyst in the body. Research has found that for people with insulin-dependent diabetes, taking an oral dose of L-alanine can be more effective than a conventional bedtime snack in preventing nighttime hypoglycemia.

102

Arginine

Arginine retards the growth of tumors and cancer by enhancing immune function. It increases the size and activity of the thymus gland, which manufactures T lymphocytes (T cells), crucial components of the immune system. Arginine may therefore benefit those suffering from AIDS and malignant diseases that suppress the immune system. It is also good for liver disorders such as cirrhosis of the liver and fatty liver; it aids in liver detoxification by neutralizing ammonia. It may reduce the effects of chronic alcohol toxicity. Seminal fluid contains arginine. Studies suggest that sexual maturity may be delayed by arginine deficiency; conversely, arginine is useful in treating sterility in men. It is found in high concentrations in the skin and connective tissues, making it helpful for healing and repair of damaged tissue.

Arginine is important for muscle metabolism. It helps to maintain a proper nitrogen balance by acting as a vehicle for transportation and storage, and aiding in the excretion, of excess nitrogen. Studies have shown that it also reduces nitrogen losses in people who have undergone surgery, and improves the function of cells in lymphatic tissue. This amino acid aids in weight loss because it facilitates an increase in muscle mass and a reduction of body fat. It is also involved in a variety of enzymes and hormones. It aids in stimulating the pancreas to release insulin, is a component of the pituitary hormone vasopressin, and assists in the release of growth hormones. Because arginine is a component of collagen and aids in building new bone and tendon cells, it can be good for arthritis and connective tissue disorders. Scar tissue that forms during wound healing is made up of collagen, which is rich in arginine. A variety of functions, including insulin production, glucose tolerance, and liver lipid metabolism, are impaired if the body is deficient in arginine.

This amino acid can be produced in the body; however, in newborn infants, production may not occur quickly enough to keep up with requirements. It is therefore deemed essential early in life. Foods high in arginine include carob, chocolate, coconut, dairy products, gelatin, meat, oats, peanuts, soybeans, walnuts, white flour, wheat, and wheat germ.

People with viral infections such as herpes should *not* take supplemental arginine, and should avoid foods rich in arginine and low in the amino acid lysine (see below), as this appears to promote the growth of certain viruses. L-Arginine supplements should be avoided by pregnant and lactating women. Persons with schizophrenia should avoid amounts over 30 milligrams daily. Long-term use, especially of high doses, is not recommended. One study found that several weeks of large doses may result in thickening and coarsening of the skin.

Asparagine

Asparagine, created from another amino acid, aspartic acid, is needed to maintain balance in the central nervous system; it prevents you from being either overly nervous or overly calm. As it is converted back into aspartic acid, asparagine releases energy that brain and nervous system cells use for metabolism. It promotes the process by which one amino acid is transformed into another in the liver.

103

Aspartic Acid

Because aspartic acid increases stamina, it is good for fatigue and depression, and plays a vital role in metabolism. Chronic fatigue may result from low levels of aspartic acid, because this leads to lowered cellular energy. In proper balance, aspartic acid is beneficial for neural and brain disorders; it has been found in increased levels in people with epilepsy and in decreased levels in people with some types of depression. It is good for athletes and helps to protect the liver by aiding in the removal of excess ammonia. Aspartic acid combines with other amino acids to form molecules that absorb toxins and remove them from the bloodstream. It helps to move certain minerals across the intestinal lining and into the blood and cells, aids cell function, and aids the function of RNA and DNA, which are the carriers of genetic information. It enhances the production of immunoglobulins and antibodies (immune system proteins). Plant protein, especially that found in sprouting seeds, contains an abundance of aspartic acid. The artificial sweetener aspartame is made from aspartic acid and phenylalanine, another amino acid.

Carnitine

Carnitine is not an amino acid in the strictest sense (it is actually a substance related to the B vitamins). However, because it has a chemical structure similar to that of amino acids, it is usually considered together with them.

Unlike true amino acids, carnitine is not used for protein synthesis or as a neurotransmitter. Its main function in the body is to help transport long-chain fatty acids, which are burned within the cells, mainly in the mitochondria, to provide energy. This is a major source of energy for the muscles. Carnitine thus increases the use of fat as an energy source. This prevents fatty buildup, especially in the heart, liver, and skeletal muscles. Carnitine may be useful in treating chronic fatigue syndrome (CFS), because a disturbance in the function of the mitochondria (the site of energy production within the cells) may be a factor in fatigue. Studies have shown decreased carnitine levels in many people with CFS.

Carnitine reduces the health risks posed by poor fat metabolism associated with diabetes; inhibits alcohol-induced fatty liver; and lessens the risk of heart disorders. Studies have shown that damage to the heart from cardiac surgery can be reduced by treatment with carnitine. According to *The American Journal of Cardiology,* one study showed that proprionyl-L-carnitine, a carnitine derivative, helps to ease the severe pain of intermittent claudication, a condition in which a blocked artery in the thigh decreases the supply of blood and oxygen to leg muscles, causing pain, especially with physical activity. Carnitine has the ability to lower blood triglyceride levels, aid in weight loss, improve the motility of sperm, and improve muscle strength in people with neuromuscular disorders. It may be useful in treating Alzheimer's disease. Conversely, carnitine deficiency may be a contributor to certain types of muscular dystrophy, and it has been shown that these disorders lead to losses of carnitine in the urine. People with such conditions need greater than normal amounts of carnitine. Carnitine also enhances the effectiveness of the antioxidant vitamins E and C. It works with antioxidants to help slow the aging process by promoting the synthesis of carnitine acetyl-transferease, an enzyme in the mitochondria of brain cells that is vital for the production of cellular energy there.

Carnitine can be manufactured by the body if sufficient amounts of iron, vitamin B_1 (thiamine), vitamin B_6 (pyridoxine), and the amino acids lysine and methionine are available. The synthesis of carnitine also depends on the presence of adequate levels of vitamin C. Inadequate intake of any of these nutrients can result in a carnitine deficiency. Carnitine can also be obtained from food, primarily meats and other foods of animal origin.

Many cases of carnitine deficiency have been identified as partly genetic in origin, resulting from an inherited defect in carnitine synthesis. Possible symptoms of deficiency include confusion, heart pain, muscle weakness, and obesity. Because of their generally greater muscle mass, men need more carnitine than women do. Vegetarians are more likely than nonvegetarians to be deficient in carnitine because it is not found in vegetable protein. Moreover, neither methionine nor lysine, two of the key constituents from which the body makes carnitine, are obtainable from vegetable sources in sufficient amounts. To ensure adequate production of carnitine, vegetarians should take supplements or should eat grains, such as cornmeal, that have been fortified with lysine.

Supplemental carnitine is available in different forms, including D-carnitine, L-carnitine, and DL-carnitine. DL-carnitine is not recommended, as it may cause toxicity. Acetyl-L-carnitine (ALC), a carnitine derivative produced naturally in the body, is involved in carbohydrate and protein metabolism and in the transport of fats into the mitochondria. It increases levels of carnitine in tissues and even surpasses the metabolic potency of carnitine. ALC has become one of the most studied compounds for its anti-aging effects, particularly with regard to degeneration of the brain and nervous system. Several major studies have shown that daily supplementation with ALC significantly slows the progression of Alzheimer's disease, resulting in less deterioration in memory, attention and language, and spatial abilities. It also can be used to treat other cognitive disorders, as well as depression.

ALC provides numerous other benefits to many of the body's systems. It helps to limit damage caused by oxygen starvation, enhance the immune system, protect against oxidative stress, stimulate the antioxidant activity of certain enzymes, protect membranes, slow cerebral aging, prevent nerve disease associated with diabetes and sciatica, modulate hormonal changes caused by physical stress, and increase the performance-enhancing benefits of branched-chain amino acids.

Total brain levels of ALC (and carnitine) decline with age. In most of the studies of ALC done with humans, subjects took 500 to 2,500 milligrams daily, in divided doses. No toxic or serious side effects have been reported.

Citrulline

The body makes citrulline from another amino acid, ornithine. Citrulline promotes energy, stimulates the immune system, is metabolized to form L-arginine, and detoxifies ammonia, which damages living cells. Citrulline is found primarily in the liver. It is helpful in treating fatigue.

Cysteine and Cystine

These two amino acids are closely related; each molecule of cystine consists of two molecules of cysteine joined together. Cysteine is very unstable and is easily converted to L-cystine; however, each form is capable of converting into the other as needed. Both are sulfur-containing amino acids that aid in the formation of skin and are important in detoxification.

Cysteine is present in alpha-keratin, the chief protein constituent of the fingernails, toenails, skin, and hair. Cysteine aids in the production of collagen and promotes the proper elasticity and texture of the skin. It is also found in a variety of other proteins in the body, including several of the digestive enzymes.

Cysteine helps to detoxify harmful toxins and protect the body from radiation damage. It is one of the best free radical destroyers, and works best when taken with selenium and vitamin E. Cysteine is also precursor to glutathione, a substance that detoxifies the liver by binding with potentially harmful substances there. It helps to protect the liver and brain from damage due to alcohol, drugs, and toxic compounds in cigarette smoke.

Since cysteine is more soluble than cystine, it is used more readily in the body and is usually best for treating most illnesses. This amino acid is formed from L-methionine in the body. Vitamin B_6, vitamin B_{12}, and folate are necessary for cysteine synthesis, which may not take place as it should in the presence of chronic disease. Therefore, people with chronic illnesses may need higher than normal doses of cysteine, as much as 1,000 milligrams three times daily for a month at a time.

Supplementation with L-cysteine is recommended in the treatment of rheumatoid arthritis, hardening of the arteries, and mutagenic disorders such as cancer. It promotes healing after surgery and severe burns, chelates heavy metals, and binds with soluble iron, aiding in iron absorption. This amino acid also promotes the burning of fat and the building of muscle. Because of its ability to break down mucus in the respiratory tract, L-cysteine is often beneficial in the treatment of bronchitis, emphysema, and tuberculosis. It promotes healing from respiratory disorders and plays an important role in the activity of white blood cells, which fight disease.

Cystine or the N-acetyl form of cysteine (N-acetylcysteine, or NAC) may be used in place of L-cysteine. NAC aids in preventing side effects from chemotherapy and radiation therapy. Because it increases glutathione levels in the lungs, kidneys, liver, and bone marrow, it has an anti-aging effect on the body—reducing the accumulation of age spots, for example. NAC has been shown to be more effective at boosting glutathione levels than supplements of cystine or even of glutathione itself.

People who have diabetes should be cautious about taking supplemental cysteine because it is capable of inactivating insulin. Persons with cystinuria, a rare genetic condition that leads to the formation of cystine kidney stones, should not take cysteine.

Gamma-Aminobutyric Acid

Gamma-aminobutyric acid (GABA) is an amino acid that acts as a neurotransmitter in the central nervous system. It is essential for brain metabolism, aiding in proper brain function. GABA is formed in the body from another amino acid, glutamic acid. Its function is to decrease neuron activity and inhibit nerve cells from overfiring. Together with niacinamide and inositol, it prevents anxiety- and stress-related messages from reaching the motor centers of the brain by occupying their receptor sites.

GABA can be taken to calm the body in much the same way as diazepam (Valium), chlordiazepoxide (Librium), and other tranquilizers, but without the fear of addiction. GABA has been used in the treatment of epilepsy and hypertension. It is good for depressed sex drive because of its ability as a relaxant. It is also useful for enlarged prostate, probably because it plays a role in the mechanism regulating the release of sex hormones. GABA is effective in treating attention deficit disorder and may reduce cravings for alcohol. It is also thought to promote growth hormone secretion.

Too much GABA, however, can cause increased anxiety, shortness of breath, numbness around the mouth, and tingling in the extremities. Further, abnormal levels of GABA unbalance the brain's message-delivery system and may cause seizures.

Glutamic Acid

Glutamic acid is an excitatory neurotransmitter that increases the firing of neurons in the central nervous system. It is a major excitatory neurotransmitter in the brain and spinal cord. It is converted into either glutamine or GABA.

This amino acid is important in the metabolism of sugars and fats, and aids in the transportation of potassium into the spinal fluid and across the blood-brain barrier. Although it does not pass the blood-brain barrier as readily as glutamine does, it is found at high levels in the blood and may infiltrate the brain in small amounts. The brain can use glutamic acid as fuel. Glutamic acid can detoxify ammonia by picking up nitrogen atoms, in the process creating another amino acid, glutamine. The conversion of glutamic acid into glutamine is the only means by which ammonia in the brain can be detoxified.

Glutamic acid helps to correct personality disorders and is useful in treating childhood behavioral disorders. It is used in the treatment of epilepsy, mental retardation, muscular dystrophy, ulcers, and hypoglycemic coma, a complication of insulin treatment for diabetes. It is a component of folate (folic acid), a B vitamin that helps the body break down amino acids. Because one of its salts is monosodium glutamate (MSG), glutamic acid should be avoided by anyone who is allergic to MSG.

Glutamine

Glutamine is the most abundant free amino acid found in the muscles of the body. Because it can readily pass the blood-brain barrier, it is known as brain fuel. In the brain, glutamine is converted into glutamic acid—which is essential for cerebral function—and vice versa. It also increases the amount of GABA, which is needed to sustain proper brain function and mental activity. It assists in maintaining the proper acid/alkaline balance in the body, and is the basis of the building blocks for the synthesis of RNA and DNA. It promotes mental ability and the maintenance of a healthy digestive tract.

When an amino acid is broken down, nitrogen is released. The body needs nitrogen, but free nitrogen can form ammonia, which is especially toxic to brain tissues. The liver can convert nitrogen into urea, which is excreted in the urine, or nitrogen may attach itself to glutamic acid. This process forms glutamine. Glutamine is unique among the amino acids in that each molecule contains not one nitrogen atom but two. Thus, its creation helps to clear ammonia from the tissues, especially brain tissue, and it can transfer nitrogen from one place to another.

Glutamine is found in large amounts in the muscles and is readily available when needed for the synthesis of skeletal muscle proteins. Because this amino acid helps to build and maintain muscle, supplemental glutamine is useful for dieters and bodybuilders. More important, it helps to prevent the kind of muscle-wasting that can accompany prolonged bed rest or diseases such as cancer and AIDS. This is because stress and injury (including surgical trauma) cause the muscles to release glutamine into the bloodstream. In fact, during times of stress, as much as one third of the glutamine present in the muscles may be released. As a result, stress and/or illness can lead to the loss of skeletal muscle. If enough glutamine is available, however, this can be prevented.

Supplemental L-glutamine can be helpful in the treatment of arthritis, autoimmune diseases, fibrosis, intestinal disorders, peptic ulcers, connective tissue diseases such as polymyositis and scleroderma, and tissue damage due to radiation treatment for cancer. L-glutamine can enhance mental functioning and has been used to treat a range of problems, including developmental disabilities, epilepsy, fatigue, impotence, depression, schizophrenia, and senility. It preserves glutathione in the liver and protects that organ from the effects of acetaminophen overdose. It enhances antioxidant protection. L-glutamine decreases sugar cravings and the desire for alcohol, and is useful for recovering alcoholics.

Many plant and animal substances contain glutamine, but it is easily destroyed by cooking. If eaten raw, spinach and parsley are good sources. Supplemental glutamine must be kept absolutely dry or the powder will degrade into ammonia and pyroglutamic acid. Glutamine should *not* be taken by persons with cirrhosis of the liver, kidney problems, Reye's syndrome, or any type of disorder that can result in an accumulation of ammonia in the blood. For such individuals, taking supplemental glutamine may only cause further damage to the body. Be aware that although the names sound similar, glutamine, glutamic acid (also sometimes called glutamate), glutathione, gluten, and monosodium glutamate are all different substances.

Glutathione

Like carnitine, glutathione is not technically one of the amino acids. It is a compound classified as a tripeptide, and the body produces it from the amino acids cysteine, glutamic acid, and glycine. Because of its close relationship to these amino acids, however, it is usually considered together with them.

111

Glutathione is a powerful antioxidant that is produced in the liver. The largest stores of glutathione are found in the liver, where it detoxifies harmful compounds so that they can be excreted through the bile. Some glutathione is released from the liver directly into the bloodstream, where it helps to maintain the integrity of red blood cells and protect white blood cells. Glutathione is also found in the lungs and the intestinal tract. It is needed for carbohydrate metabolism and appears to exert anti-aging effects, aiding in the breakdown of oxidized fats that may contribute to atherosclerosis. It can mitigate some of the damage caused by tobacco smoke because it modifies the harmful effects of aldehydes, chemicals present in cigarette smoke that damage cells and molecules, and it may protect the liver from alcohol-induced damage.

A deficiency of glutathione first affects the nervous system, causing such symptoms as lack of coordination, mental disorders, tremors, and difficulty maintaining balance. These problems are believed to be due to the development of lesions in the brain. A study sponsored in part by the National Cancer Institute found that people with HIV disease who had low glutathione levels had a lower survival rate over a three-year period than those whose glutathione levels were normal. As we age, glutathione levels decline, although it is not known whether this is because we use it more rapidly or produce less of it to begin with. Unfortunately, if not corrected, the lack of glutathione in turn accelerates the aging process.

Supplemental glutathione is expensive, and the effectiveness of oral formulas is questionable. To raise glutathione levels, it is better to supply the body with the raw materials it uses to make this compound: cysteine, glutamic acid, and glycine. The N-acetyl form of cysteine, N-acetylcysteine (NAC), is considered particularly effective for this purpose.

Glycine

Glycine retards muscle degeneration by supplying additional creatine, a compound that is present in muscle tissue and is utilized in the construction of DNA and RNA. It improves glycogen storage, thus freeing up glucose for energy needs. Glycine is essential for the synthesis of nucleic acids, bile acids, and other nonessential amino acids in the body. It is used in many gastric antacid agents. Because high concentrations of glycine are found in the skin and connective tissues, it is useful for repairing damaged tissues and promoting healing.

Glycine is necessary for central nervous system function and a healthy prostate. It functions as an inhibitory neurotransmitter and as such can help prevent epileptic seizures. It has been used in the treatment of manic (bipolar) depression, and can also be effective for hyperactivity.

Having too much of this amino acid in the body can cause fatigue, but having the proper amount produces more energy. If necessary, glycine can be converted into the amino acid serine in the body.

Histidine

Histidine is an essential amino acid that is significant in the growth and repair of tissues. It is important for the maintenance of the myelin sheaths, which protect nerve cells, and is needed for the production of both red and white blood cells. Histidine also protects the body from radiation damage, helps lower blood pressure, aids in removing heavy metals from the system, and may help in the prevention of AIDS.

Histidine levels that are too high may lead to stress and even psychological disorders such as anxiety and schizophrenia; people with schizophrenia have been found to have high levels of histidine in their bodies. Inadequate levels of histidine may contribute to rheumatoid arthritis and may be associated with nerve deafness. Methionine has the ability to lower histidine levels.

Histamine, an important immune system chemical, is derived from histidine. Histamine aids in sexual arousal. Because the availability of histidine influences histamine production, taking supplemental histidine—together with vitamins B_3 (niacin) and B_6 (pyridoxine), which are required for the transformation from histidine to histamine—may help improve sexual functioning and pleasure. Because histamine also stimulates the secretion of gastric juices, histidine may be helpful for people with indigestion resulting from a lack of stomach acid.

Persons with manic (bipolar) depression should not take supplemental histidine unless a deficiency has been identified. Natural sources of histidine include rice, wheat, and rye.

Homocysteine

Homocysteine is an amino acid that is produced in the body in the course of methionine metabolism. This amino acid has been the focus of increasing attention in recent years, because high levels of homocysteine in the blood are associated with an increased risk of cardiovascular disease. Further, it is known that homocysteine has a toxic effect on cells lining the arteries, makes the blood more prone to clotting, and promotes the oxidation of low-density lipoproteins (LDL, the so-called "bad cholesterol"), which makes it more likely that cholesterol will be deposited as plaque in the blood vessels.

Like other amino acids, homocysteine does perform a necessary function in the body. It is then usually broken down quickly into the amino acid cysteine and other important compounds, including adenosine triphosphate (ATP, an important source of cellular energy) and S-adenosylmethionine (SAMe). However, a genetic defect or, more commonly, deficiencies of vitamins B_6 and B_{12} and folate (folic acid) can prevent homocysteine from converting rapidly enough. As a result, high levels of the amino acid accumulate in the body, damaging cell membranes and blood vessels, and increasing the risk of cardiovascular disease, particularly atherosclerosis. Vitamins B_6 and B_{12} and folate work together to facilitate the breakdown of homocysteine, and thus help protect against heart disease.

Isoleucine

Isoleucine, one of the essential amino acids, is needed for hemoglobin formation and also stabilizes and regulates blood sugar and energy levels. It is metabolized in muscle tissue. It is one of the three branched-chain amino acids. These amino acids are valuable for athletes because they enhance energy, increase endurance, and aid in the healing and repair of muscle tissue.

Isoleucine has been found to be deficient in people suffering from many different mental and physical disorders. A deficiency of isoleucine can lead to symptoms similar to those of hypoglycemia.

Food sources of isoleucine include almonds, cashews, chicken, chickpeas, eggs, fish, lentils, liver, meat, rye, most seeds, and soy protein. It is also available in supplemental form. Supplemental L-isoleucine should always be taken with a correct balance of the other two branched-chain amino acids, L-leucine and L-valine—approximately 2 milligrams each of leucine and valine for each milligram of isoleucine. Combination supplements that provide all three of the branched-chain amino acids are available and may be more convenient to use.

Leucine

Leucine is an essential amino acid and one of the branched-chain amino acids (the others are isoleucine and valine). These work together to protect muscle and act as fuel. They promote the healing of bones, skin, and muscle tissue, and are recommended for those recovering from surgery. Leucine also lowers elevated blood sugar levels and aids in increasing growth hormone production.

Natural sources of leucine include brown rice, beans, meat, nuts, soy flour, and whole wheat. Supplemental L-leucine must be taken in balance with L-isoleucine and L-valine (*see* Isoleucine in this section), and it should be taken in moderation, or symptoms of hypoglycemia may result. An excessively high intake of leucine may also contribute to pellagra, and may increase the amount of ammonia present in the body.

Lysine

Lysine is an essential amino acid that is a necessary building block for all protein. It is needed for proper growth and bone development in children; it helps calcium absorption and maintains a proper nitrogen balance in adults. This amino acid aids in the production of antibodies, hormones, and enzymes, and helps in collagen formation and tissue repair. Because it helps to build muscle protein, it is good for those recovering from surgery and sports injuries. It also lowers high serum triglyceride levels.

Another very useful ability of this amino acid is its capacity for fighting cold sores and herpesviruses. Taking supplemental L-lysine, together with vitamin C with bioflavonoids, can effectively fight and/or prevent herpes outbreaks, especially if foods containing the amino acid arginine are avoided. Supplemental L-lysine also may decrease acute alcohol intoxication.

Lysine is an essential amino acid, and so cannot be manufactured in the body. It is therefore vital that adequate amounts be included in the diet. Deficiencies can result in anemia, bloodshot eyes, enzyme disorders, hair loss, an inability to concentrate, irritability, lack of energy, poor appetite, reproductive disorders, retarded growth, and weight loss. Food sources of lysine include cheese, eggs, fish, lima beans, milk, potatoes, red meat, soy products, and yeast.

Methionine

Methionine is an essential amino acid that assists in the breakdown of fats, thus helping to prevent a buildup of fat in the liver and arteries that might obstruct blood flow to the brain, heart, and kidneys. The synthesis of the amino acids cysteine and taurine may depend on the availability of methionine. This amino acid helps the digestive system; helps to detoxify harmful agents such as lead and other heavy metals; helps diminish muscle weakness, prevent brittle hair, and protect against radiation; and is beneficial for people with osteoporosis or chemical allergies. It is useful also in the treatment of rheumatic fever and toxemia of pregnancy.

Methionine is a powerful antioxidant. It is a good source of sulfur, which inactivates free radicals and helps to prevent skin and nail problems. It is also good for people with Gilbert's syndrome, an anomaly of liver function, and is required for the synthesis of nucleic acids, collagen, and proteins found in every cell of the body. It is beneficial for women who take oral contraceptives because it promotes the excretion of estrogen. It reduces the level of histamine in the body, which can be useful for people with schizophrenia, whose histamine levels are typically higher than normal.

As levels of toxic substances in the body increase, the need for methionine increases. The body can convert methionine into the amino acid cysteine, a precursor of glutathione. Methionine thus protects glutathione; it helps to prevent glutathione depletion if the body is overloaded with toxins. Since glutathione is a key neutralizer of toxins in the liver, this protects the liver from the damaging effects of toxic compounds.

An essential amino acid, methionine is not synthesized in the body and so must be obtained from food sources or from dietary supplements. Good food sources of methionine include beans, eggs, fish, garlic, lentils, meat, onions, soybeans, seeds, and yogurt. Because the body uses methionine to derive a brain food called choline, it is wise to supplement the diet with choline or lecithin (which is high in choline) to ensure that the supply of methionine is not depleted.

Ornithine

Ornithine helps to prompt the release of growth hormone, which promotes the metabolism of excess body fat. This effect is enhanced if ornithine is combined with arginine and carnitine. Ornithine is necessary for proper immune-system and liver function. This amino acid also detoxifies ammonia and aids in liver regeneration. High concentrations of ornithine are found in the skin and connective tissue, making it useful for promoting healing and repairing damaged tissues.

Ornithine is synthesized in the body from arginine, and in turn serves as the precursor of citrulline, proline, and glutamic acid. Supplemental L-ornithine should *not* be taken by children, pregnant women, nursing mothers, or anyone with a history of schizophrenia, unless they are specifically directed to do so by a physician.

Phenylalanine

117

Phenylalanine is an essential amino acid. Because it can cross the blood-brain barrier, it can have a direct effect on brain chemistry. Once in the body, phenylalanine can be converted into another amino acid, tyrosine, which in turn is used to synthesize two key neurotransmitters that promote alertness: dopamine and norepinephrine. Because of its relationship to the action of the central nervous system, this amino acid can elevate mood, decrease pain, aid in memory and learning, and suppress the appetite. It can be used to treat arthritis, depression, menstrual cramps, migraines, obesity, Parkinson's disease, and schizophrenia.

Phenylalanine is available in three different forms, designated L-, D-, and DL-. The L- form is the most common type and is the form in which phenylalanine is incorporated into the body's proteins. The D- type acts as a painkiller. The DL- form is a combination of the D- and the L-. Like the D- form, it is effective for controlling pain, especially the pain of arthritis; like the L- form, it functions as a building block for proteins, increases mental alertness, suppresses the appetite, and helps people with Parkinson's disease. It has been used to alleviate the symptoms of premenstrual syndrome (PMS) and various types of chronic pain.

Supplemental phenylalanine, as well as products containing aspartame (an artificial sweetener made from phenylalanine and another amino acid, aspartic acid) should *not* be taken by pregnant women or by people who suffer from anxiety attacks, diabetes, high blood pressure, phenylketonuria (PKU), or preexisting pigmented melanoma, a type of skin cancer.

Proline

Proline improves skin texture by aiding in the production of collagen and reducing the loss of collagen through the aging process. It also helps in the healing of cartilage and the strengthening of joints, tendons, and heart muscle. It works with vitamin C to promote healthy connective tissue. Proline is obtained primarily from meat sources, dairy products, and eggs.

Serine

Serine is needed for the proper metabolism of fats and fatty acids, the growth of muscle, and the maintenance of a healthy immune system. It is a component of brain proteins and the protective myelin sheaths that cover nerve fibers. It is important in RNA and DNA function, cell membrane formation, and creatine synthesis. It also aids in the production of immunoglobulins and antibodies. However, too-high serine levels in the body may have adverse effects on the immune system.

Serine can be made from glycine in the body, but this process requires the presence of sufficient amounts of vitamins B_3 and B_6 and folic acid. Food sources of serine include meat and soy foods, as well as many foods that often cause allergic reactions, such as dairy products, wheat gluten, and peanuts. It is included as a natural moisturizing agent in many cosmetics and skin care preparations.

Taurine

High concentrations of taurine are found in the heart muscle, white blood cells, skeletal muscle, and central nervous system. It is a building block of all the other amino acids as well as a key component of bile, which is needed for the digestion of fats, the absorption of fat-soluble vitamins, and the control of serum cholesterol levels. Taurine can be useful for people with atherosclerosis, edema, heart disorders, hypertension, or hypoglycemia. It is vital for the proper utilization of sodium, potassium, calcium, and magnesium, and it has been shown to play a particular role in sparing the loss of potassium from the heart muscle. This helps to prevent the development of potentially dangerous cardiac arrhythmias.

Taurine has a protective effect on the brain, particularly if the brain is dehydrated. It is used to treat anxiety, epilepsy, hyperactivity, poor brain function, and seizures. Taurine is found in concentrations up to four times greater in the brains of children than in those of adults. It may be that a deficiency of taurine in the developing brain is involved in seizures. Zinc deficiency also is commonly found in people with epilepsy, and this may play a part in the deficiency of taurine. Taurine is also associated with zinc in maintaining eye function; a deficiency of both may impair vision. Taurine supplementation may benefit children with Down syndrome and muscular dystrophy. This amino acid is also used in some clinics for breast cancer treatment.

Excessive losses of taurine through the urine can be caused by many metabolic disorders. Cardiac arrhythmias, disorders of platelet formation, intestinal problems, an overgrowth of candida, physical or emotional stress, a zinc deficiency, and excessive consumption of alcohol are all associated with high urinary losses of taurine. Excessive alcohol consumption also causes the body to lose its ability to utilize taurine properly. Taurine supplementation may reduce symptoms of alcohol withdrawal. Diabetes increases the body's requirements for taurine; conversely, supplementation with taurine and cystine may decrease the need for insulin.

Taurine is found in eggs, fish, meat, and milk, but not in vegetable proteins. It can be synthesized from cysteine in the liver and from methionine elsewhere in the body, as long as sufficient quantities of vitamin B_6 are present. For vegetarians, synthesis by the

119

body is crucial. For individuals with genetic or metabolic disorders that prevent the synthesis of taurine, taurine supplementation is required.

Threonine

Threonine is an essential amino acid that helps to maintain the proper protein balance in the body. It is important for the formation of collagen, elastin, and tooth enamel, and aids liver and lipotropic function when combined with aspartic acid and methionine. A precursor of the amino acids glycine and serine, threonine is present in the heart, central nervous system, and skeletal muscle, and helps to prevent fatty buildup in the liver. It enhances the immune system by aiding in the production of antibodies, and may be helpful in treating some types of depression.

Because the threonine content of grains is low, vegetarians are more likely than others to have deficiencies.

Tryptophan

Tryptophan is an essential amino acid that is necessary for the production of vitamin B_3 (niacin). It is used by the brain to produce serotonin, a necessary neurotransmitter that transfers nerve impulses from one cell to another and is responsible for normal sleep. Consequently, tryptophan helps to combat depression and insomnia and to stabilize moods. It helps to control hyperactivity in children, alleviates stress, is good for the heart, aids in weight control by reducing appetite, and enhances the release of growth hormone. It is good for migraine headaches and may reduce some of the effects of nicotine. Sufficient amounts of vitamins B_6 (pyridoxine) and C, folate, and magnesium are necessary for the formation of tryptophan, which, in turn, is required for the formation of serotonin. A study reported in the *Archives of General Psychiatry* found that women with a history of bulimia nervosa, an eating disorder, experienced relapses after they took an amino acid mixture lacking tryptophan. Researchers believe that insufficient tryptophan altered brain serotonin levels and, consequently, the transmission of nerve impulses. A lack of tryptophan and magnesium may contribute to coronary artery spasms.

The best dietary sources of tryptophan include brown rice, cottage cheese, meat, peanuts, and soy protein. This amino acid is not available in supplement form in the United States. In November of 1989, the U.S. Centers for Disease Control (CDC) reported evidence linking L-tryptophan supplements to a blood disorder called eosinophilia-myalgia syndrome (EMS). Several hundred cases of this illness—which is characterized by an elevated white blood cell count and can also cause such symptoms as fatigue, muscular pain, respiratory ailments, edema, and rash—were reported. After the CDC established an association between the blood disorder and products containing L-tryptophan in New Mexico, the U.S. Food and Drug Administration (FDA) first warned consumers to stop taking L-tryptophan supplements, then recalled all products in which L-tryptophan was the sole or a major component. Subsequent research showed that it was contaminants in the supplements, *not* the tryptophan, that was probably responsible for the problem, but tryptophan supplements are still banned from the market in the United States. According to the FDA, at least thirty-eight deaths were attributable to the tryptophan supplements.

Tyrosine

Tyrosine is important to overall metabolism. It is a precursor of adrenaline and the neurotransmitters norepinephrine and dopamine, which regulate mood and stimulate metabolism and the nervous system. Tyrosine acts as a mood elevator; a lack of adequate amounts of tyrosine leads to a deficiency of norepinephrine in the brain, which in turn can result in depression. It also acts as a mild antioxidant, suppresses the appetite, and helps to reduce body fat. It aids in the production of melanin (the pigment responsible for skin and hair color) and in the functions of the adrenal, thyroid, and pituitary glands. It is also involved in the metabolism of the amino acid phenylalanine.

Tyrosine attaches to iodine atoms to form active thyroid hor-

121

mones. Not surprisingly, therefore, low plasma levels of tyrosine have been associated with hypothyroidism. Symptoms of tyrosine deficiency can also include low blood pressure, low body temperature (such as cold hands and feet), and restless leg syndrome.

Supplemental L-tyrosine has been used for stress reduction, and research suggests it may be helpful against chronic fatigue and narcolepsy. It has been used to help individuals suffering from anxiety, depression, low sex drive, allergies, and headaches, as well as persons undergoing withdrawal from drugs. It may also help people with Parkinson's disease.

Natural sources of tyrosine include almonds, avocados, bananas, dairy products, lima beans, pumpkin seeds, and sesame seeds. Tyrosine can also be produced from phenylalanine in the body. Supplements of L-tyrosine should be taken at bedtime or with a high-carbohydrate meal so that it does not have to compete for absorption with other amino acids.

Persons taking monoamine oxidase (MAO) inhibitors, commonly prescribed for depression, must strictly limit their intake of foods containing tyrosine and should *not* take any supplements containing L-tyrosine, as it may lead to a sudden and dangerous rise in blood pressure. Anyone who takes prescription medication for depression should discuss necessary dietary restrictions with his or her physician.

Valine

Valine, an essential amino acid, has a stimulant effect. It is needed for muscle metabolism, tissue repair, and the maintenance of a proper nitrogen balance in the body. Valine is found in high concentrations in muscle tissue. It is one of the branched-chain amino acids, which means that it can be used as an energy source by muscle tissue. It may be helpful in treating liver and gallbladder disease, and it is good for correcting the type of severe amino acid deficiencies that can be caused by drug addiction. An excessively high level of valine may lead to such symptoms as a crawling sensation in the skin and even hallucinations.

Dietary sources of valine include dairy products, grains, meat, mushrooms, peanuts, and soy protein. Supplemental L-valine should always be taken in balance with the other branched-chain amino acids, L-isoleucine and L-leucine (*see* Isoleucine in this section).

SIX

Antioxidants

INTRODUCTION

Antioxidants are natural compounds that help protect the body from harmful free radicals. These are atoms or groups of atoms that can cause damage to cells, impairing the immune system and leading to infections and various degenerative diseases such as heart disease and cancer. Antioxidants therefore play a beneficial role in the prevention of disease. Free radical damage is thought by scientists to be the basis for the aging process as well. (*See* Free Radicals on page 125.)

There are a number of known free radicals that occur in the body, the most common of which are oxygen-derived free radicals, such as superoxide radicals and hydroxyl radicals, hypochlorite radicals, hydrogen peroxide, various lipid peroxides, and nitric oxide. They may be formed by exposure to radiation, including exposure to the sun's rays; exposure to toxic chemicals such as those found in cigarette smoke, polluted air, and industrial and household chemicals; and various metabolic processes, such as the process of breaking down stored fat molecules for use as an energy source.

Free radicals are normally kept in check by the action of *free radical scavengers* that occur naturally in the body. These scavengers neutralize the free radicals. Certain enzymes serve this vital function. Four important enzymes that neutralize free radicals are

FREE RADICALS

A free radical is an atom or group of atoms that contains at least one unpaired electron. Electrons are negatively charged particles that usually occur in pairs, forming a chemically stable arrangement. If an electron is unpaired, another atom or molecule can easily bond with it, causing a chemical reaction. Because they join so readily with other compounds, free radicals can effect dramatic changes in the body, and they can cause a lot of oxidative damage. Each free radical may exist for only a tiny fraction of a second, but the damage it leaves behind can be irreversible, particularly damage to heart muscle cells, nerve cells, and certain immune system sensor cells.

Free radicals are normally present in the body in small numbers. Biochemical processes naturally lead to the formation of free radicals, and under normal circumstances the body can keep them in check. Indeed, not all free radicals are bad. Free radicals produced by the immune system destroy viruses and bacteria. Other free radicals are involved in producing vital hormones and activating enzymes that are needed for life. We need free radicals to produce energy and various substances that the body requires. If there is excessive free radical formation, however, damage to cells and tissues can occur. The formation of a large number of free radicals stimulates the formation of more free radicals, leading to even more damage.

Many different factors can lead to an excess of free radicals. Exposure to radiation, whether from the sun or from medical x-rays, activates the formation of free radicals, as does exposure to environmental pollutants such as tobacco smoke and automobile exhaust. Diet also can contribute to the formation of

continued on next page

superoxide dismutase (SOD), methionine reductase, catalase, and glutathione peroxidase. The body makes these as a matter of course. There are also a number of phytochemicals and nutrients that act as antioxidants, including vitamin A, beta-carotene and other carotenoids, flavonoids, vitamins C and E, and the mineral selenium. Another antioxidant is the hormone melatonin, which is a powerful free radical neutralizer. Certain herbs have antioxidant properties as well.

continued from previous page
free radicals. When the body obtains nutrients through the diet, it utilizes oxygen and these nutrients to create energy. In this oxidation process, oxygen molecules containing unpaired electrons are released. These oxygen free radicals can cause damage to the body if produced in extremely large amounts. A diet that is high in fat can increase free radical activity because oxidation occurs more readily in fat molecules than it does in carbohydrate or protein molecules. Cooking fats at high temperatures, particularly frying foods in oil, can produce large numbers of free radicals.

The presence of a dangerous number of free radicals can alter the way in which the cells code genetic material. Changes in protein structure can occur as a result of errors in protein synthesis. The body's immune system may then see this altered protein as a foreign substance and try to destroy it. The formation of mutated proteins can eventually damage the immune system and lead to leukemia and other types of cancer, as well as to many other diseases.

In addition to damaging genetic material, free radicals can destroy the protective cell membranes. Calcium levels in the body may be upset as well. Over time, the body produces more free radicals than it does scavengers. The resulting imbalance is what causes us to age.

Substances known as antioxidants neutralize free radicals by binding to their free electrons. Antioxidants available in supplement form include the enzymes superoxide dismutase and glutathione peroxidase; vitamin A, beta-carotene, and vitamins C and E; the minerals selenium and zinc; and the hormone melatonin. By destroying free radicals, antioxidants help to detoxify and protect the body.

Although many antioxidants can be obtained from food sources such as sprouted grains and fresh fruits and vegetables, it is difficult to get enough of them from these sources to hold back the free radicals constantly being generated in our polluted environment. We can minimize free radical damage by taking supplements of key nutrients. A high intake of antioxidant nutrients appears to be especially protective against cancer.

Antioxidants work synergistically in giving protection against free radical damage, so it is better to take smaller doses of several different antioxidants than a large amount of only one. For example, while beta-carotene by itself is an excellent antioxidant, a mix of natural carotenoids provides more health benefits than beta-carotene alone. There are many good combination formulas available that make it easy to take multiple antioxidants every day.

THE ANTIOXIDANTS

Alpha-Lipoic Acid

Alpha-lipoic acid (ALA) is a powerful antioxidant—both on its own and as a "recycler" of vitamin E and vitamin C. It can restore the antioxidant properties of these vitamins after they have neutralized free radicals. ALA also stimulates the body's production of glutathione and aids in the absorption of coenzyme Q_{10}, both important antioxidants. Because ALA is soluble in both water and fat, it can move into all parts of cells to deactivate free radicals.

Supplemental ALA has been used for almost three decades in Europe to treat peripheral nerve degeneration and to help control blood sugar levels in people with diabetes. It also helps to detoxify the liver of metal pollutants, block cataract formation, protect nerve tissues against oxidative stress, and reduce blood cholesterol levels. According to Lester Packer, Ph.D., Professor of Molecular and Cell Biology at the University of California—Berkeley and a leading antioxidant researcher, ALA could play an important role in the prevention and treatment of chronic degenerative diseases such as diabetes and cardiovascular disease. ALA is known also as a metabolic antioxidant, because without it, cells cannot use sugar to produce energy. The body does not produce large amounts of ALA, and since it is found primarily in only a few foods, including spinach, broccoli, and organ meats, supplementation may be necessary.

Bilberry

The herb bilberry (*Vaccinium myrtillus*), a European relative of the American blueberry, contains natural antioxidants that keep capillary walls strong and flexible. They also help to maintain the flexibility of the walls of red blood cells and allow them to pass through the capillaries better. Bilberry contains anthocyanidins, phytochemicals that help to lower blood pressure, inhibit clot formation, and enhance blood supply to the nervous system. Studies indicate that anthocyanidins can provide up to fifty times the antioxidant protection of vitamin E and ten times the protection of vitamin C. In addition, this herb protects the eyes and may enhance vision; supports and strengthens collagen structures; inhibits the growth of bacteria; acts as an anti-inflammatory; and has anti-aging and anticarcinogenic effects. Tests have shown that the compound glucoquinine, found in bilberry leaves, helps to lower blood sugar levels.

Burdock

The herb burdock (*Arctium lappa*) was tested by researchers at the Chia Nan College of Pharmacy and Science in Taiwan for its antioxidant properties. They found that burdock is a powerful antioxidant, capable of scavenging hydrogen peroxide and superoxide radicals. It also showed a marked scavenging effect against hydroxyl radicals. The study showed also that burdock and vitamin E quench more free radicals when used in combination. Burdock also protects against cancer by helping to control cell mutation.

Carotenoids

See under Vitamin A and the Carotenoids.

Coenzyme Q₁₀

Coenzyme Q_{10} is an antioxidant that is structurally similar to vitamin E. It plays a crucial role in the generation of cellular energy, is a significant immunologic stimulant, increases circulation, has anti-aging effects, and is beneficial for the cardiovascular system. Also known as *ubiquinone* (from *quinone,* a type of coenzyme, and *ubiquitous,* because it exists everywhere in the body), coenzyme Q_{10} is found in highest concentrations in the heart, followed by the liver, kidney, spleen, and pancreas. Within the mitochondria, the cells' energy-production centers, coenzyme Q_{10} helps to metabolize fats and carbohydrates. It also helps to maintain the flexibility of cell membranes.

In Japan, coenzyme Q_{10} has been approved for use in treating congestive heart failure. Various research reports suggest that coenzyme Q_{10} also may be beneficial in treating cancer, AIDS, muscular dystrophy, allergies, gastric ulcers, myopathy, periodontal disease, diabetes, and deafness.

Curcumin (Turmeric)

Found in the spice turmeric, the phytochemical curcumin has antioxidant properties that prevent the formation of and neutralize existing free radicals. It stops precancerous changes within DNA and interferes with enzymes necessary for cancer progression. Curcumin stops the oxidation of cholesterol, thus protecting against the formation of plaque in the arteries. In a study of chronic smokers, those who took curcumin excreted a substantially lower level of mutagens (substances that induce cells to mutate) in their urine, a reflection of how well the body is dealing with these cancer-causing substances. Curcumin also blocks toxic compounds from reaching or reacting with body tissues, and may prevent cataracts.

Curcumin should not be taken by anyone who has biliary tract obstruction or is taking anticoagulants, as curcumin stimulates bile secretion and acts as a blood-thinner.

Flavonoids

Flavonoids are especially potent antioxidants and metal chelators. They are chemical compounds that plants produce to protect themselves from parasites, bacteria, and cell injury. More than 4,000 chemically unique flavonoids are known; they occur in fruits, vegetables, spices, seeds, nuts, flowers, and bark. Wine (particularly red wine), apples, blueberries, bilberries, onions, soy products, and tea are some of the best food sources of flavonoids. Certain flavonoids in fruits and vegetables have much greater antioxidant activity than vitamins C and E or beta-carotene. In fact, flavonoids protect the antioxidant vitamins from oxidative damage.

Numerous medicinal herbs contain therapeutic amounts of flavonoids; they often are a major component of an herb's medicinal activity.

Garlic

This versatile healing herb also has antioxidant properties. The sulfhydryl (sulfur and hydrogen) compounds in garlic are potent chelators of toxic heavy metals, binding with them so that they can be excreted. These same compounds are effective protectants against oxidation and free radicals. Garlic aids in the detoxification of peroxides such as hydrogen peroxide and helps to prevent fats from being oxidized and deposited in tissues and arteries. Garlic also contains antioxidant nutrients such as vitamins A and C and selenium.

Studies on aged garlic extract (AGE) have shown that the aging process substantially boosts garlic's antioxidant potential. AGE protects against DNA damage, keeps blood vessels healthy, and guards against radiation and sunlight damage. According to researcher and nutritionist Robert I-San Lin, Ph.D., aged garlic extract can prevent liver damage caused by carbon tetrachloride, a common indoor pollutant and free radical generator. Overall, aged garlic supplements provide a greater concentration of garlic's beneficial compounds. If you're worried about "garlic breath" putting a strain on your social life, choose an odorless and tasteless form such as Kyolic aged garlic extract from Wakunaga of America. Aged garlic extract reduces blood cholesterol levels, thus lowering the risk of heart attack; provides protection from heart disease by preventing clots that can lead to heart attacks and strokes; and helps lower high blood pressure.

Ginkgo Biloba

Ginkgo biloba is an herb with powerful antioxidant effects in the brain, retina, and cardiovascular system. It is well known for its ability to enhance circulation, and a study reported in the *Journal of the American Medical Association* showed that it has a measurable effect on dementia in people with Alzheimer's disease and people recovering from strokes. Other studies indicate that it can improve both long- and short-term memory, and enhance concentration. Gingko biloba has also been used to treat hearing problems, impotence, and macular degeneration.

Anyone who takes prescription anticoagulant (blood-thinning) medication or who uses over-the-counter painkillers regularly should consult a health care provider before using gingko biloba, as the combination may result in internal bleeding.

Glutathione

Glutathione is a protein that is produced in the liver from the amino acids cysteine, glutamic acid, and glycine. It is a powerful antioxidant that inhibits the formation of, and protects against cellular damage from, free radicals. It helps to defend the body against damage from cigarette smoking, exposure to radiation, cancer chemotherapy, and toxins such as alcohol. As a detoxifier of heavy metals and drugs, it aids in the treatment of blood and liver disorders.

Glutathione protects cells in several ways. It neutralizes oxygen molecules before they can harm cells. Together with selenium, it forms the enzyme glutathione peroxidase, which neutralizes hydrogen peroxide. It is also a component of another antioxidant enzyme, glutathione-S-transferase, which is a broad-spectrum liver-detoxifying enzyme.

Glutathione protects not only individual cells but also the tissues of the arteries, brain, heart, immune cells, kidneys, lenses of the eyes, liver, lungs, and skin against oxidant damage. It plays a role in preventing cancer, especially liver cancer, and may actually target carcinogens, make them water-soluble, and then help escort them from the body. It may also have an anti-aging effect. The rate at which we age is directly correlated with reduced concentrations of glutathione in cellular fluids; as we grow older, glutathione levels drop, resulting in a decreased ability to deactivate free radicals.

Glutathione can be taken in supplement form. The production of glutathione by the body can be boosted by taking supplemental dehydroepiandrosterone (DHEA), a hormone; N-acetylcysteine

131

or L-cysteine; and L-methionine. Studies suggest that this may be a better way of raising glutathione levels than taking glutathione itself.

Grape Seed Extract

See under Oligomeric Proanthocyanidins in this section.

Green Tea

Green tea contains compounds known as polyphenols, including phytochemicals that have antioxidant, antibacterial, antiviral, and health-enhancing properties. Tests on epigallocatechin gallate (EGCG), a particular type of polyphenol in green tea, have shown that it is able to penetrate the body's cells and shield DNA from hydrogen peroxide, a potent free radical. Green tea protects against cancer, lowers cholesterol levels, and reduces the clotting tendency of the blood. It also shows promise as a weight-loss aid that can promote the burning of fat and help to regulate blood sugar and insulin levels.

Green tea is simply the dried leaves of the tea plant. Black tea undergoes natural fermentation, which converts tannins, astringent phytochemicals, into more complex compounds. This fermentation process destroys most of black tea's polyphenols, rendering it less effective as an antioxidant.

Melatonin

The hormone melatonin is an efficient free radical scavenger and singlet oxygen quencher. Singlet oxygen is an "excited" oxygen molecule whose excessive discharge of energy causes damage to other body molecules. While most antioxidants work only in certain parts of certain cells, melatonin can permeate any cell in any part of the body. More important, melatonin is one of the few antioxidants that can penetrate the mitochondria, the cells' "power plants," which produce energy. Melatonin does seem to protect the mitochondria from free radical damage. In laboratory experiments, melatonin supplementation has been found to extend the lifespan of mice. Other nonhuman laboratory studies have shown that supplemental melatonin can inhibit cancer growth, help modulate the immune system, and protect against degenerative diseases. Melatonin also stimulates the enzyme glutathione peroxidase, another antioxidant.

Methionine

A unique amino acid, methionine neutralizes hydroxyl radicals, one of the most dangerous types of free radicals. Most often a byproduct of reactions between heavy metals and less toxic free radicals, hydroxyl radicals can be formed also during strenuous exercise or exposure to high levels of radiation, and can damage any type of body tissue.

N-Acetylcysteine (NAC)

The sulfur-containing amino acid cysteine is needed to produce the free radical fighter glutathione and to help maintain it at adequate levels in the cells. N-acetylcysteine (NAC) is a more stable form of cysteine that can be taken in supplement form.

NAC is used by the liver and the lymphocytes to detoxify chemicals and other poisons. It is a powerful detoxifier of alcohol, tobacco smoke, and environmental pollutants, all of which are immune suppressors. Taking supplemental NAC can boost the levels of protective enzymes in the body, thus slowing some of the cellular damage that is characteristic of aging. NAC supplementation may also decrease both the frequency and duration of infectious diseases. It has been used to treat AIDS and chronic bronchitis.

People with diabetes should not take supplemental NAC without first consulting a health care provider, as it can interfere with the effectiveness of insulin.

Nicotinamide Adenine Dinucleotide (NADH)

Also known as coenzyme 1, nicotinamide adenine dinucleotide with high-energy hydrogen, or NADH, is the "spark" that ignites energy production in the body's cells. NADH's high antioxidant capacity derives from its ability to reduce levels of substances. NADH plays a central role in DNA repair and maintenance, and in the cellular immune defense system. Studies report that NADH also can inhibit the auto-oxidation of the neurotransmitter dopamine, which causes the release of toxic chemicals that may damage sensitive parts of the brain.

Oligomeric Proanthocyanidins

Oligomeric proanthocyanidins (OPCs) are naturally occurring substances present in a variety of food and botanical sources. They are unique phytochemicals known as flavonoids that have powerful antioxidant capabilities. OPCs are highly water soluble, so the body is able to absorb them rapidly. Clinical tests suggest that OPCs may be as much as fifty times more potent than vitamin E and twenty times more potent than vitamin C in terms of bioavailable antioxidant activity. What's more, OPCs work with the antioxidant glutathione to recycle and restore oxidized vitamin C, thus increasing the vitamin's effectiveness. Because they are able to cross the blood-brain barrier, OPCs can protect the brain and spinal nerves against free radical damage. In addition to their antioxidant activity, OPCs protect the liver from damage caused by toxic doses of acetaminophen, a nonprescription pain reliever; they strengthen and repair connective tissue, including that of the cardiovascular system; and they support the immune system and slow aging. They also moderate allergic and inflammatory responses by reducing histamine production.

OPCs are found throughout plant life; however, the two main sources are pine bark extract (Pycnogenol), produced from the French maritime pine tree, and grape seed extract, made from the seeds of the wine grape (*Vitis vinifera*). Pycnogenol was the first source of OPCs discovered, and the process for extracting it was patented in the 1950s. Pycnogenol is a trademarked name for pine bark extract, not a generic term for OPCs from other sources.

Pycnogenol

See under Oligomeric Proanthocyanidins in this section.

Selenium

Selenium is an essential trace mineral that functions as an antioxidant in partnership with vitamin E to protect tissues and cell membranes. Among other things, it increases antioxidant enzyme levels in cells. Selenium is also an integral component of the antioxidant enzyme glutathione peroxidase (each molecule of this enzyme contains four atoms of selenium). Glutathione peroxidase targets harmful hydrogen peroxide in the body and converts it into water. It is a particularly important guardian of blood cells and of the heart, liver, and lungs.

Numerous plants contain selenium, including garlic, asparagus, and grains, but the levels depend on soil content, which varies from one geographic region to another.

Use caution when taking supplemental selenium. Amounts higher than 1,000 micrograms (1 milligram) daily may be toxic.

Silymarin

Extracted from the seeds of the herb milk thistle, silymarin has been used for centuries to treat liver disease. The active ingredients in milk thistle are several types of flavonoids (powerful antioxidants), known collectively as silymarin. Silymarin guards the liver from oxidative damage. It also protects the liver from toxins, drugs, and the effects of alcohol, and promotes the growth of new liver cells. In addition, silymarin increases levels of glutathione, a potent antioxidant enzyme produced in the liver.

Superoxide Dismutase

Superoxide dismutase (SOD) is an enzyme. SOD revitalizes cells and reduces the rate of cell destruction. It neutralizes the most common, and possibly the most dangerous, free radicals—superoxide radicals. Superoxide radicals instigate the breakdown of synovial fluid, the lubricant for the body's joints. This leads to friction and, ultimately, inflammation. SOD works synergistically with the enzyme catalase, which is abundant throughout the body. Catalase removes hydrogen peroxide byproducts created by SOD reactions.

SOD also aids in the body's utilization of zinc, copper, and manganese. Its levels tend to decline with age, while free radical production increases. Its potential as an anti-aging treatment is currently being explored.

Chemically speaking, there are two forms of this enzyme. The copper/zinc form (known as Cu/Zn SOD) exerts its antioxidant properties in the cytoplasm of cells. This is the watery fluid that surrounds all the other cellular components. Metabolic activity that takes place in the cytoplasm results in the production of free radicals; Cu/Zn neutralizes them. The manganese form (Mn SOD) is active in the mitochondria, structures within cells where energy is produced. The production of cellular energy also leads to the creation of free radicals.

SOD occurs naturally in barley grass, broccoli, Brussels sprouts, cabbage, wheatgrass, and most green plants. It is also available in supplement form. SOD supplements in pill form must be enteric coated—that is, coated with a protective substance that allows the pill to pass intact through the stomach acid into the small intestines to be absorbed. Cell Guard from Biotec Food Corporation and KAL SOD-3 from Nutraceutical International Corporation are good sources of SOD.

Vitamin A and the Carotenoids

A class of phytochemicals, carotenoids are fat-soluble pigments found in yellow, red, green, and orange vegetables and fruits. They are a potent family of antioxidants that include alpha-carotene, beta-carotene, lycopene, lutein, and zeaxanthin. Of the more than 500 carotenoids found in nature, about 50 can be converted into vitamin A in the body.

Carotenoids quench singlet oxygen, which is not, chemically speaking, a free radical, but is nevertheless highly reactive and can damage body molecules. Carotenoids also act as anticancer agents, decrease the risk of cataracts and age-related macular degeneration, and inhibit heart disease. Studies have shown that carotenoids found in tomato juice (lycopene), carrots (alpha- and beta-carotene) and spinach (lutein) may help to protect against cancer by reducing oxidative and other damage to DNA.

Together, the antioxidants alpha-lipoic acid, coenzyme Q_{10}, vitamin C, and vitamin E help conserve carotenoids in tissues.

The body converts beta-carotene into vitamin A as needed. Any leftover beta-carotene then acts as an antioxidant, breaking free radical chain reactions and preventing the oxidation of cholesterol. It reduces the oxidation of DNA and disables reactive oxygen species molecules generated by exposure to sunlight and air pollution, preventing damage to eyes, lungs, and skin.

A recent laboratory study found that taking high doses of supplemental of beta-carotene alone (50,000 international units or more daily) may interfere with the normal control of cell division. It is best to take a carotenoid complex containing a variety of carotenoids.

Vitamin C

Vitamin C is a very powerful antioxidant that also recharges other antioxidants, such as vitamin E, to keep them potent. Its water solubility makes it an efficient free radical scavenger in body fluids. Some studies have shown that vitamin C is the first line of antioxidant defense in plasma against many different kinds of free radicals. The cells of the brain and spinal cord, which frequently incur free radical damage, can be protected by significant amounts of vitamin C. This vitamin also guards against atherosclerosis by preventing damage to artery walls. Vitamin C acts as a more potent free radical scavenger in the presence of the phytochemical hesperidin.

Vitamin E

Vitamin E is a powerful antioxidant that prevents the oxidation of lipids (fats). Fat oxidation has been implicated in the process that leads to atherosclerosis. Vitamin E is fat soluble and, since cell membranes are composed of lipids, it effectively prevents the cells' protective coatings from becoming rancid as a result of the assault of free radicals. Vitamin E also improves oxygen utilization, enhances immune response, plays a role in the prevention of cataracts caused by free radical damage, and may reduce the risk of coronary artery disease.

The natural form of vitamin E (d-alpha tocopherol) is superior to the synthetic version (dl-alpha tocopherol). New evidence suggests that zinc is needed to maintain normal blood concentrations of vitamin E. Selenium enhances vitamin E uptake. These two nutrients work together in the body.

Zinc

Zinc's main antioxidant function is in the prevention of fat oxidation. In addition, it is a constituent of the antioxidant enzyme superoxide dismutase (SOD). Zinc is also needed for proper maintenance of vitamin E levels in the blood and aids in the absorption of vitamin A.

Combination Antioxidant Supplements

No single antioxidant protects all body systems; rather, each one has protective properties for particular body parts or functions. Products that combine two or more of these vital nutrients are available. You can easily find formulas that give you a balance of multiple antioxidants. Some recommended antioxidant combination products include the following:

- ACES + Zinc and ACES + Selenium from Carlson Laboratories.
- Advanced Carotenoid Complex from Solgar.
- Body Language Super Antioxidant from OxyFresh USA.
- Cell Guard from Biotec Food Corporation.
- Glutathione Booster from Carlson Laboratories.
- Juice Plus from Kelco.
- Life Guard from Thompson Nutritional Products.
- Oxy-5000 Forte from American Biologics.
- Revenol from Neways, Inc.

Using a combination supplement is often more convenient than taking many different products separately.

Enzymes

INTRODUCTION

The late Dr. Edward Howell, a physician and pioneer in enzyme research, called enzymes the "sparks of life." These energized protein molecules play a necessary role in virtually all of the biochemical activities that go on in the body. They are essential for digesting food, for stimulating the brain, for providing cellular energy, and for repairing all tissues, organs, and cells. Life as we know it could not exist without the action of enzymes, even in the presence of sufficient amounts of vitamins, minerals, water, and other nutrients.

In their primary role, enzymes are catalysts—substances that accelerate and precipitate the hundreds of thousands of biochemical reactions in the body that control life's processes. If it were not for the catalytic action of enzymes, most of these reactions would take place far too slowly to sustain life. Enzymes are not consumed in the reactions they facilitate.

Each enzyme has a specific function in the body that no other enzyme can fulfill. The chemical shape of each enzyme is specialized so that it can initiate a reaction only in a certain substance, or in a group of closely related substances, and not in others. The substance on which an enzyme acts is called the *substrate*. Because there must be a different enzyme for every substrate, the body must produce a great number of different enzymes.

THE FUNCTIONS OF ENZYMES

Enzymes assist in practically all bodily functions. Digestive enzymes break down food particles for storage in the liver or muscles. This stored energy is later converted by other enzymes for use by the body when necessary. Iron is concentrated in the blood by the action of enzymes; other enzymes in the blood help the blood to coagulate in order to stop bleeding. Uricolytic enzymes catalyze the conversion of uric acid into urea. Respiratory enzymes aid in eliminating carbon dioxide from the lungs. Enzymes assist the kidneys, liver, lungs, colon, and skin in removing wastes and toxins from the body. Enzymes also utilize the nutrients ingested by the body to construct new muscle tissue, nerve cells, bone, skin, and glandular tissue. One enzyme can take dietary phosphorus and convert it into bone. Enzymes prompt the oxidation of glucose, which creates energy for the cells. Enzymes also protect the blood from dangerous waste materials by converting these substances to forms that are easily eliminated by the body. Indeed, the functions of enzymes are so many and so diverse that it would be impossible to name them all.

Enzymes are often divided into two groups: digestive enzymes and metabolic enzymes. Digestive enzymes are secreted along the gastrointestinal tract and break down foods, enabling the nutrients to be absorbed into the bloodstream for use in various bodily functions. There are three main categories of digestive enzymes: amylase, protease, and lipase. Amylase, found in saliva and in the pancreatic and intestinal juices, breaks down carbohydrates. It begins to act as soon as you start chewing (this is why it is important to chew your food well). Different types of amylase break down specific types of sugars. For example, lactase breaks down lactose (milk sugar), maltase breaks down maltose (malt sugar), and sucrase breaks down sucrose (cane and beet sugar). Protease, found in the stomach juices and also in the pancreatic and intestinal juices, helps to digest protein. Lipase, found in the stomach and pancreatic juices, and also present in fats in foods, aids in fat digestion. Another component of the digestive process is hydrochloric acid. While not technically an enzyme itself, it interacts with digestive enzymes as they perform their functions.

Metabolic enzymes are enzymes that catalyze the various chemical reactions within the cells, such as energy production and detoxification. The activities of all of the body's organs, tissues, and cells are governed by metabolic enzymes. They are the workers that build the body from proteins, carbohydrates, and fats. Metabolic enzymes are found doing their specific work in the blood, organs, and tissues. Each body tissue has its own specific set of metabolic enzymes.

Two particularly important metabolic enzymes are superoxide dismutase (SOD) and its partner, catalase. SOD is an antioxidant that protects the cells by attacking a common free radical, superoxide. (*See* Superoxide Dismutase in chapter six—ANTIOXIDANTS.) Catalase breaks down hydrogen peroxide, a metabolic waste product, and liberates oxygen for the body to use.

Of the tens of thousands of enzymes needed, the body uses more of its enzyme-producing potential to produce the two dozen enzymes that control the breakdown and utilization of proteins, fats, and carbohydrates than it uses to create the hundreds of metabolic enzymes necessary to maintain the rest of the tissues and organs in their functions.

141

FOOD ENZYMES

While the body manufactures a supply of enzymes, it can also obtain enzymes from food. Unfortunately, enzymes are extremely sensitive to heat. Even low to moderate heat (118°F or above) destroys most enzymes in food, so to obtain enzymes from the diet, one must eat raw foods. Eating raw foods or, alternatively, taking enzyme supplements, helps prevent depletion of the body's own enzymes and thus reduces the stress on the body.

Enzymes can be found in many different foods, from both plant and animal sources. Avocados, papayas, pineapples, bananas, and mangos are all high in enzymes. Sprouts are the richest source. Unripe papaya and pineapple are excellent sources of enzymes. The enzymes extracted from papaya and pineapple—papain and bromelain, respectively—are proteolytic enzymes, which break down proteins.

Many fat-containing foods also supply lipase, which breaks down fats. In fact, fat in food exposed only to pancreatic lipase (the lipase produced by the body) in the intestines is not as well digested as fat that is first worked on in the stomach by food lipase. Pancreatic lipase digests fat in a highly alkaline environment (the intestines), whereas lipase found in food fats works in a more acidic environment (the stomach). The optimal extraction of nutrients from fats depends on the work of different fat-digesting enzymes in successive stages.

Hydrochloric acid (HCl) comes in several different forms, including lysine HCl and betaine HCl. Betaine HCl is derived from sugar beets. When new, HCl capsules and tablets are almost white in color, but sometimes they can turn a deep purple color when they age. Supplemental HCl is not sold in powder or liquid form because contact with the teeth can damage tooth enamel. HCl has a sulfur-like odor.

Superoxide dismutase occurs naturally in a variety of food sources, including alfalfa, barley grass, broccoli, Brussels sprouts, cabbage, wheatgrass, and most dark green plants.

As powerful as they are, enzymes cannot act alone. They require adequate amounts of other substances, known as coenzymes, to be fully active. Among the most important coenzymes are the B-complex vitamins, vitamin C, vitamin E, and zinc.

COMMERCIALLY AVAILABLE ENZYMES

The majority of commercially available enzymes are digestive enzymes extracted from various sources. (Scientists are unable to manufacture enzymes synthetically.) Most commercial enzyme products are made from animal enzymes, such as pancreatin and pepsin, which help in the digestion of food once it has reached the lower stomach and the intestinal tract. Some companies make their supplements from enzymes extracted from aspergillus, a type of fungus. These enzymes begin their predigestive work in the upper stomach. All of these products are used primarily to aid the digestion of foods and absorption of nutrients, especially protein.

If proteins are not completely digested, undigested protein particles may make their way into the bloodstream through the intestinal wall with other nutrients. This phenomenon is known as *leaky gut syndrome,* and it can result in allergic reactions that may be more or less severe, depending upon the strength of the immune system. This is one reason why the proper digestion of proteins is so important.

Any enzyme that acts on protein and prepares it for absorption is called a proteolytic enzyme. Proteolytic enzymes available in supplement form include pepsin, trypsin, rennin, pancreatin, and chymotrypsin. In addition to aiding digestion, proteolytic enzymes have been shown to be beneficial as anti-inflammatory agents. Pancreatin, derived from secretions of animal pancreas, is a focus of cancer research, because people with cancer are often deficient in this enzyme. Pancreatin is used in the treatment of digestive problems, viral infections, and sports injuries, as well as pancreatic insufficiency, food allergies, cystic fibrosis, autoimmune disorders, and other chronic illnesses.

Also available in supplement form are the antioxidant enzymes superoxide dismutase (SOD) and catalase.

The following table lists some common enzymes and their substrates.

Enzyme	Substrate
Amylase	Carbohydrates
Bromelain	Proteins
Cellulase	Fiber
Chymopapain	Proteins
Diastase	Carbohydrates
Glucoamylase	Carbohydrates
Hemicellulase	Carbohydrates
Hyaluronidase	Proteins, adhesions, fibrin
Invertase	Carbohydrates
Lactase	Lactose (milk sugar)
Lipase	Fats
Maltase	Carbohydrates

Enzyme	Substrate
Pancreatin	Proteins, fats, carbohydrates
Papain	Proteins, fats, carbohydrates
Pectinase	Carbohydrates
Pepsin	Proteins
Phytase	Carbohydrates
Plasmin	Proteins
Protease	Proteins
Rennin	Proteins
Trypsin	Proteins

Enzyme supplements may not be for everyone, however. During pregnancy, it is a rule to be careful with supplements in general. Nursing mothers also should be careful about supplements, to avoid affecting their milk. People who have hemophilia or who take anticoagulants (blood-thinners) should consult their health care providers before taking large amounts of enzymes. Anyone contemplating surgery where there is high risk of bleeding should ask his or her physician for advice before taking any supplement.

WHAT'S ON THE SHELVES

Enzymes are available over the counter in tablet, capsule, powder, and liquid forms. They may be sold in combination with each other or as separate items. Some enzyme products also contain garlic to aid digestion.

For maximum benefit, any digestive enzyme supplement you choose should contain all of the major enzyme groups—amylase, protease, and lipase. Digestive enzymes should be taken after meals, unless you are eating processed and/or cooked foods, in which case it is best to take them during the meal. You can make your own digestive enzymes by drying papaya seeds, placing them in a pepper grinder, and sprinkling them on your foods. These have a peppery taste.

If you take supplemental superoxide dismutase, make sure to choose a product that is enteric coated—that is, coated with a protective substance that allows the SOD to pass intact through the stomach acid to be absorbed in the small intestine. Do not crush or chew these pills. All forms of enzymes should be kept in a reasonably cool place to insure potency because they are susceptible to moisture.

Research has shown that as we grow older, the body's ability to produce enzymes decreases. At the same time, malabsorption of nutrients, tissue breakdown, and chronic health conditions increase. Taking supplemental enzymes can help to ensure that you continue to get the full nutritional value from your foods. We believe that enzyme supplementation is vital for elderly persons.

The following are a few recommended enzyme complex products:

- AbsorbAid from Nature's Sources is made from plant enzymes and includes lipase, amylase, and protease from bromelain, as well as cellulase and lactase. It has been shown to significantly improve the absorption of nutrients, especially essential fatty acids and zinc.

- Acid-Ease from Prevail Corporation is a digestive aid from natural plant sources that includes amylase, lipase, and cellulase, as well as the soothing herbs marshmallow root and slippery elm.
- All Complete Enzymes from TriMedica, Inc. is a blend of plant enzymes that provide a full range of essential enzymes, plus coenzymes for added effectiveness. It is designed to adapt to various body temperatures and pH levels without losing potency. Ingredients include amylase, lipase, bromelain, papain, protease, cellulase, acidophilus, bifidus, and trace minerals.
- Bio-Gestin from Biotec Foods (a division of AgriGenic Food Corporation) is freeze-dried mature green papaya containing papain and chymopapain. The naturally sweet taste of the papaya makes these especially good capsules to open and sprinkle over food before eating.
- Bio-Zyme from Metagenics contains proteolytic enzymes, including chymotrypsin, trypsin, and raw pancreas concentrate, enteric coated for absorption in the intestines so that they may benefit inflammatory conditions.

- Cardio Enzyme Formula from Prevail Corporation contains a combination of enzymes, herbs, and nutrients, including protease 1 and 2, amylase, cellulase, and lipase; extracts of hawthorn berry, dan-shen root, arjun bark, passionflower, ginkgo leaf, ginkgo rhizome, and garlic; and magnesium, vitamin B_6, vitamin B_{12}, folic acid, vitamin C, taurine, L-carnitine, and L-lysine, all in a special blend to support the heart.
- Cholesterol Enzyme Formula from Prevail Corporation is an enzyme and antioxidant formula designed to promote cardiovascular health. Ingredients include pantothenic acid, beta-glycan, guggul, gamma-oryzanol, garlic, cellulase, amylase, protease 1 and 2, and lipase 2.
- D.A. #34 Food Enzymes from Carlson Laboratories contains pancreatin and ox bile, with enough capability in each tablet to digest 34 grams of protein, 120 grams of carbohydrates, and 21 grams of fat. Ox bile is a beneficial supplement for people with gallbladder disorders.
- Daily Essential Enzymes from Source Naturals is a full-spectrum digestive enzyme supplement containing protease (acid stable), lipase, amylase, cellulase, and lactase. The powder in the capsules has very little taste of its own, and the contents may be added to food that is not hot (over 110°F) by sprinkling over food (this is a good option for vegetarians who want to avoid gelatin capsules). This supplement is designed to work in both the acidic environment of the stomach and the more alkaline environment of the intestines.
- Digest Support from Natrol is a multi-enzyme formula containing all three classes of digestive enzymes (proteolytic, amyolytic, and lipolytic), including protease 1 and 2, amylase, cellulase, lipase, maltase, and sucrase. It also contains A-galactosidase, an enzyme that acts on galactose, a breakdown product of lactose (milk sugar), and fights gas.
- Elastase from Cardiovascular Research contains elastase, a proteolytic enzyme found in pancreatic juices.
- Infla-Zyme Forte from American Biologics is a combination of enzymes and antioxidants for people requiring supplemental digestive enzymes to aid in the breakdown of proteins, fats,

and carbohydrates. It may also be helpful for chronic or acute inflammation. Its ingredients include amylase, bromelain, catalase, chymotrypsin, L-cysteine, lipase, pancreatin, papain, rutin, superoxide dismutase, trypsin, and zinc. If taken as a digestive aid, the recommended dosage is 1 to 3 tablets following each meal; if you use it for other purposes, such as illness, inflammation, and/or injury, take 3 to 6 tablets one hour before each meal or between meals. Infla-Zyme Forte may be taken by persons on sodium-restricted diets.

- Inflazyme from Ecological Formulas is a blend of bromelain and vitamin C.

- Lipothiamine from Cardiovascular Research contains a specially prepared form of vitamin B_1 (thiamine) plus lipoate (thioctic acid), both enzyme cofactors involved in the production of cellular energy.

- Mega-Zyme from Enzymatic Therapy is an extra-strength pancreatic and digestive enzyme tablet. Each tablet contains protease, amylase, lipase, trypsin, papain, bromelain, and lysozyme.

- MegaZymes from MegaFood is a vegetarian enzyme and herbal formula made from plant-based enzymes, including amylase, cellulase, glucoamylase, invertase, lactase, lipase, and protease, blended with the tonic herbs caraway, gentian, and ginger, plus acidophilus to support healthy intestinal flora.

- Metazyme from Metagenics is a plant-derived enzyme supplement that contains protease, amylase, lipase, and cellulase.

- Multi-Zyme from FoodScience Laboratories of Vermont is an enteric-coated tablet containing pepsin, bromelain, ox bile, pancreas extract, papain, proteases, amylase, lipases, cellulase, and hydrochloric acid (HCl). HCl is another component of the digestive process that works with enzymes to break down foods.

- Serraflazyme from Cardiovascular Research contains serrapeptase (serratio peptidase), a proteolytic enzyme with anti-inflammatory properties.

- Vegetarian Enzyme Complex from Futurebiotics contains protease, amylase, celluase, lipase, papain, and bromelain.

- Wobenzym N from Marlyn Nutraceuticals contains a combination of enzymes designed to interact synergistically with each other. Its ingredients include bromelain, chymotrypsin, pancreatin, papain, rutin, and trypsin.

Other sources for quality enzyme supplements include the National Enzyme Company and Miller Pharmacal Group. Miller Pharmacal products, available through health care professionals only, include:

- Milcozyme, a two-part enzyme supplement with glutamic acid HCl, betaine HCl, papain, pepsin, and an enteric-coated side of the same tablet with pancreatin, lipase, amylase, and bromelain.
- Carbozyme, which contains betaine HCl, trypsin, chymotrypsin, bromelain, pancreatin, mannitol, thymus extract, lipase, amylase, and papain.
- Proteolytic Enzymes, made with enteric-coated trypsin and chymotrypsin.
- Karbozyme (not to be confused with the sound-alike product above), which contains pancreatin, sodium bicarbonate, and potassium bicarbonate.
- MM-Zyme, which contains pancreatic lipase, bromelain, amylase, raw pancreas extract, papain, trypsin, chymotrypsin, and selenium.

Finally, while not technically an enzyme product, Bioperine 10 from Nature's Plus also enhances the digestion and absorption of nutrients. It contains an extract of black pepper (*Piper nigrum*), and when taken with food or with vitamin, mineral, or herbal supplements, it helps food to digest and accelerates the distribution of nutrients throughout the body.

Natural Food Supplements

INTRODUCTION

Natural food supplements include a wide variety of products. Almost all health food stores carry them, and a number of drug stores and supermarkets stock them on their shelves as well. In general, natural food supplements are composed of, derived from, or byproducts of foods that provide health benefits. In some cases, health benefit claims made by manufacturers are based upon a supplement's use in traditional healing; in other cases, they are based on modern scientific research.

Food supplements can be high in certain nutrients, contain active ingredients that aid digestive or metabolic processes, or provide a combination of nutrients and active ingredients. It is important to point out that some unscrupulous manufacturers make false promises. It is therefore vital to be an informed consumer. It is also necessary to be aware that many conservative "watchdog" organizations point to these few unsubstantiated products and label the whole industry as unreliable. This occurs in spite of the fact that many natural food supplements have been known to work for years; these products are medically endorsed only when they are "discovered" by researchers deemed acceptable by these groups. Such recent discoveries include garlic, aloe vera, fiber, and fish oils—substances that have been used for centuries in many parts of the world.

WHAT'S ON THE SHELVES

Food supplements come in many shapes and forms—tablets, capsules, powders, liquids, jellies, creams, biscuits, wafers, granules, and more. Product packaging depends entirely on the nature of the food supplement's composition. The potency of these products varies. Because they are made up of perishable foods, food derivatives, or food byproducts, their potency may be affected by the length of time they sit on a shelf or by the temperature at which they are kept. If you don't understand how a product is to be used, ask questions or read the available literature on the particular supplement.

If you have never used a natural food supplement, you may be uncomfortable about buying and using one for the first time. This is normal. Keep in mind that once you become familiar with its use and benefits, you won't give the idea of using it a second thought.

150

Acidophilus

See Lactobacillus Acidophilus in this section.

Adenosine Triphosphate (ATP)

Adenosine triphosphate (ATP) is a compound that serves as the immediate source of energy for the body's cells, notably muscle cells. It increases energy and stamina, builds muscular density, increases muscular strength, buffers lactic-acid buildup (the reason for sore, achy muscles after physical activity), delays fatigue, and preserves muscle fibers. ATP is produced naturally in the body from adenine, a nitrogen-containing compound; ribose, a type of sugar; and phosphate units, each containing one phosphorus atom and four oxygen atoms. ATP from Integrated Health is a good source of supplemental ATP.

Alfalfa

One of the most mineral-rich foods known, alfalfa has roots that grow as much as 130 feet into the earth. Alfalfa is available in liquid extract form and is good to use while fasting because of its chlorophyll and nutrient content. It contains calcium, magnesium, phosphorus, potassium, plus virtually all known vitamins. The minerals are in a balanced form, which promotes absorption. These minerals are alkaline, but have a neutralizing effect on the intestinal tract.

If you need a mineral supplement, alfalfa is a good choice. It has helped many arthritis sufferers. Alfalfa, wheatgrass, barley, and spirulina, all of which contain chlorophyll, have been found to aid in the healing of intestinal ulcers, gastritis, liver disorders, eczema, hemorrhoids, asthma, high blood pressure, anemia, constipation, body and breath odor, bleeding gums, infections, burns, athlete's foot, and cancer.

Aloe Vera

This plant is known for its healing effect and is used in many cosmetic and hair care products. There are over 200 different species of aloe that grow in dry regions around the world.

Aloe vera is commonly known as a skin healer, moisturizer, and softener. It is dramatically effective on burns of all types, and is also good for cuts, insect stings, bruises, acne and blemishes, poison ivy, welts, skin ulcers, and eczema. Taken internally, 98- or 99-percent pure aloe vera is known to aid in the healing of stomach disorders, ulcers, constipation, hemorrhoids, rectal itching, colitis, and all colon problems. It can also be helpful against infections, varicose veins, skin cancer, and arthritis, and is used in the treatment of AIDS.

We have had excellent results using colon cleansers containing psyllium husks in combination with aloe vera juice. We have found this combination to be good for food allergy and colon disorder sufferers. Psyllium keeps the folds and pockets in the colon free of toxic material that gathers there. The aloe vera not only has a healing effect, but if constipation or diarrhea is present, it will return the stools to normal. It takes a few weeks to cleanse the colon, but regular, periodic use will keep the colon clean. As with any substance, it is possible to develop an intolerance to aloe vera juice and/or psyllium husks, so this treatment should not be used on an ongoing basis.

Barley Grass

Barley grass is high in calcium, iron, all the essential amino acids, chlorophyll, flavonoids, vitamin B_{12}, vitamin C, and many minerals, plus enzymes. This food heals stomach, duodenal, and colon disorders as well as pancreatitis, and is an effective anti-inflammatory.

Bee Byproducts

See Bee Pollen, Bee Propolis, Honey, and Royal Jelly, all in this section.

Bee Pollen

Bee pollen is a powderlike material that is produced by the anthers of flowering plants and gathered by bees. It is composed of 10 to 15 percent protein and also contains B-complex vitamins, vitamin C, essential fatty acids, enzymes, carotene, calcium, copper, iron, magnesium, potassium, manganese, sodium, plant sterols, and simple sugars.

Like other bee products, bee pollen has an antimicrobial effect. In addition, it is useful for combating fatigue, depression, cancer, and colon disorders. It is also helpful for people with allergies because it strengthens the immune system.

It is best to obtain bee pollen from a local source, as this increases its antiallergenic properties. Fresh bee pollen should not cling together or form clumps, and it should be sold in a tightly sealed container. Some people (an estimated 0.05 percent of the population) may be allergic to bee pollen. It is best to try taking a small amount at first and watch for a developing rash, wheezing, discomfort, or any other signs of a reaction. If such symptoms occur, discontinue taking bee pollen.

Bee Propolis

Bee propolis is a resinous substance collected from various plants by bees. Bees use propolis, together with beeswax, in the construction of hives. As a supplement, it is an excellent aid against bacterial infections. Bee propolis is believed to stimulate phago-cytosis, the process by which some white blood cells destroy bacteria.

Propolis is beneficial as a salve for abrasions and bruises because of its antibacterial effect. Good results have been reported on the use of propolis against inflammation of the mucous membranes of the mouth and throat, dry cough and throat, halitosis, tonsillitis, ulcers, and acne, and for the stimulation of the immune system.

Be sure that any bee products you use smell and taste fresh. All bee products should be in tightly sealed containers. It is best to purchase these products from a manufacturer who specializes in bee products. If you are using bee products for allergies, it is best to obtain products that are produced within a ten-mile radius of your home. This way, you get a minute dose of pollen to desensitize you to the local pollen in the area.

Beta-1,3-Glucan

Beta-1,3-glucan is a polysaccharide (a complex type of carbohydrate molecule) with immune-stimulating properties. Specifically, it stimulates the activity of macrophages, immune cells that destroy cellular debris, microorganisms, and abnormal cells by surrounding and digesting them. Beta-1,3-D-glucan is a supplemental form of beta-1,3-glucan made from the cell walls of baker's yeast. Despite its origin, it does not contain any yeast proteins. It is useful for treating many bacterial, viral, and fungal diseases. It can also kill tumor cells and increase bone-marrow production. Because of its ability to protect the immune system, beta-1,3-D-glucan may protect against the effects of aging. Studies done as early as the 1970s, have found that it can reduce the size of cancerous tumors in rats. Further investigation has shown beta-1,3-D-glucan to be a potent agent for healing sores and ulcers in women who have undergone mastectomies.

153

Bifidobacterium Bifidum

Bifidobacterium bifidum aids in the synthesis of the B vitamins by creating healthy intestinal flora. *B. bifidum* is the predominant organism in the intestinal flora and establishes a healthy environment for the manufacture of the B-complex vitamins and vitamin K.

When you take antibiotics, the "friendly" bacteria in your digestive tract are destroyed along with the harmful bacteria. Supplementing your diet with *B. bifidum* helps you maintain healthy intestinal flora. Unhealthy flora can result in the liberation of abnormally high levels of ammonia as protein-containing foods are digested. This irritates the intestinal membranes. In addition, the ammonia is absorbed into the bloodstream and must be detoxified by the liver, or it will cause nausea, a decrease in appetite, vomiting, and other toxic reactions. By promoting the proper digestion of foods, the friendly bacteria also aid in preventing digestive disorders such as constipation and gas, as well as food allergies. If digestion is poor, the activity of intestinal bacteria on undigested food may lead to excessive production of the body chemical histamine, which triggers allergic symptoms.

Yeast infections of the vaginal tract respond very favorably to douching with *B. bifidum* preparations. These microorganisms destroy the pathogenic organisms. When used as an enema, *B. bifidum* also helps establish a healthy intestinal environment. It improves bowel function by aiding peristalsis, and results in the production of a softer, smoother stool. Harmful bacteria are kept in check, and toxic wastes that have accumulated in the intestines are destroyed and/or eliminated from the body.

B. bifidum has proved useful in the treatment of cirrhosis of the liver and chronic hepatitis; by improving digestion, it reduces the strain on the liver. Many people who do not respond to *L. acidophilus* react positively to *B. bifidum*. Many experts consider *B. bifidum* to be preferable to *L. acidophilus* for children and for adults with liver disorders.

Bifidus

See Bifidobacterium Bifidum in this section.

Bovine Cartilage

Cleaned, dried, and powdered bovine cartilage is a supplement that helps accelerate wound healing and reduce inflammation.

Like shark cartilage, it has been shown to be helpful for psoriasis, all types of arthritis, and ulcerative colitis. VitaCarte from Phoenix BioLabs contains pure bovine cartilage from range-raised, hormone-free cattle. Another cartilage supplement, shark cartilage, is also available, and may be preferred by some individuals.

Brewer's Yeast
See Yeast in this section.

Cellulose
See under Fiber in this section.

Cerasomal-cis-9-cetylmyristoleate
This is a modified version of a medium-chain fatty acid, cetylmyristoleate, which is found in nuts, vegetables, and animal tissue. It appears to be a very promising development in arthritis research. Studies in laboratory rats have shown it to have anti-inflammatory effects, and early clinical studies in people suggest it may be beneficial for many with osteoarthritis, rheumatoid arthritis, and psoriatic arthritis, as well as psoriasis. It is believed to work by normalizing the functioning of the immune system and reducing the production of pro-inflammatory prostaglandins.

155

While this supplement is often referred to simply as CMO, that is actually a trademarked name for a cerasomal-cis-9-cetylmyristoleate product, not a generic term. A good source of this supplement is CM+ from Metabolic Response Modifiers.

Chlorella
Chlorella is a tiny, single-celled water-grown alga containing a nucleus and an enormous amount of readily available chlorophyll. It also contains protein (approximately 58 percent), carbohydrates, all of the B vitamins, vitamins C and E, amino acids, and rare trace minerals. In fact, it is virtually a complete food. It contains more vitamin B_{12} than liver does, plus a considerable amount of beta-carotene. It has a strong cell wall, however, which makes it difficult to gain access to its nutrients. Consequently, it requires factory processing to be effective.

Chlorella is one of the few edible species of water-grown algae. The chlorophyll in chlorella can help speed the cleansing of the bloodstream. Chlorella is very high in RNA and DNA, and has been found to protect against the effects of ultraviolet radiation. Studies show that chlorella is an excellent source of protein, especially for people who cannot or who choose not to eat meat.

Chlorophyll

See under Chlorella and "Green Drinks" in this section.

Chondroitin Sulfate

Chondroitin sulfate is an important element in the creation of cartilage, the tough yet flexible connective tissue found in the joints, where it acts as a cushion, and in other parts of the body, such as the tip of the nose and the outer ear. Chemically, chondroitins belong to a group of substances classified as *glycosaminoglycans* (also referred to as *mucopolysaccharides*), which are complex types of carbohydrate molecules. Glycosaminoglycans in turn attach to proteins such as collagen and elastin, forming even more complex substances designated *proteoglycans,* which are a vital component of cartilage tissue. Chondroitin sulfate attracts water to the proteoglycans and holds it there, which is important for maintaining healthy joint cartilage. It can also protect existing cartilage from premature degeneration by blocking certain enzymes that destroy cartilage and prevent nutrients from being transported to the cartilage for repair.

Taking supplemental chondroitin sulfate, usually derived from powdered shark cartilage or cow-trachea cartilage, has been shown to be helpful in the treatment of osteoarthritis. Many times it is used in conjunction with glucosamine for even more effective therapy. The supplements are usually taken together in pill form. Neither chondroitin sulfate nor glucosamine has shown any toxic effects, but there are potential side effects for certain people. The Arthritis Foundation recommends exercising caution in taking these supplements for treatment of osteoarthritis. You should let your physician know you are taking these supplements, and discuss any allergies or potential reactions. Use caution in taking chondroitin sulfate if you are taking anticoagulants (blood-thinners) or daily aspirin, as it is chemically similar to the blood-thinner heparin. Pregnant women should not take these supplements, as there has not been sufficient study regarding their safety and potential side effects during pregnancy.

Twinlab manufactures a number of good products containing chondroitin sulfate. Glucosamine Chondroitin Sulfate from Only Natural, Inc. is a good combination source of glucosamine and chondroitin sulfate.

Citrin

Citrin is a trademarked name for a standardized herbal extract from the fruit of the *Garcinia cambogia* plant, also known as Indian berry. It inhibits the synthesis of fatty acids in the liver, promotes the burning of body fat as fuel, and suppresses the appetite. Its primary usefulness is in treating obesity, although it may also aid in preventing or slowing atherosclerosis and heart disease. It does not affect the nervous system or cause any known side effects. Citrin is an ingredient in a number of different products sold by various manufacturers.

Coenzyme A

Coenzyme A, a substance manufactured by body cells from pantotheic acid (vitamin B_5), is at the center of the whole metabolic process. It performs a vital role in the process by which the cells generate energy from glucose. Indeed, it helps produce around 90 percent of the energy the body needs to function. Coenzyme A also begins the metabolism of fatty acids. A lack of sufficient coenzyme A can result in stiff, sore muscles and a decrease in energy. Taken as a supplement, coenzyme A increases energy, supports the manufacture of substances critical for the brain and adrenal glands, helps with the manufacture of connective tissue, and supports the immune system. Studies suggest that coenzyme A may be as, if not more, beneficial than coenzyme Q_{10}.

Coenzyme Q_{10}

Coenzyme Q_{10} is present in the mitochondria of all the cells in the body. It is vital because it carries into the cells the energy-laden protons and electrons that are used to produce adenosine triphosphate (ATP), the immediate source of cellular energy (*see* Adenosine Triphosphate [ATP] on page 150). This is a constant process because the body can store only a small quantity of ATP at any one time. It is believed that as many as 75 percent of people over fifty may be deficient in coenzyme Q_{10}. A lack of sufficient coenzyme Q_{10} can lead to cardiovascular disease because without it, the heart does not have not enough energy to circulate the blood effectively.

Colloidal Silver

Colloidal silver is an inexpensive healing agent and disinfectant that has a myriad of applications. It is a clear golden liquid composed of 99.9-percent pure silver particles approximately 0.001 to 0.01 microns ($^1/_{1,000,000}$ to $^1/_{100,000}$ millimeter) in diameter that are suspended in pure water. Colloidal silver can be mixed with either tap or distilled water and applied topically, taken by mouth, or administered intravenously.

Topically, it can be used to fight fungal infections of the skin or nails and to promote the healing of burns, wounds, cuts, rashes, and sunburn. It can be used on toothaches and mouth sores, as eyedrops, and as a gargle to fight tooth decay and bad breath. It can also be used as sterilizer and can even be sprayed on air-conditioning filters and air ducts and vents to prevent germs from growing. Taken internally, colloidal silver can be used to fight infection. It has been shown to be effective against more than 650 disease-causing organisms, including *Escherichia coli* (*E. coli*) bacteria and the fungus *Candida albicans*.

Micronic Silver from Lifestar Millennium is a good source of colloidal silver. Cold Combat! from TriMedica, Inc. is a combination of sublingual forms of colloidal silver, colloidal copper, zinc, and the homeopathic remedies *Cinnabaris* and *Rhus toxicodendron*. It is good for fighting colds and flu.

Colostrum

Colostrum is a thin, yellowish fluid secreted by the mammary glands of mammalian mothers in the first days after giving birth, before the production of true milk begins. It contains high levels of protein and growth factors, as well as immune factors that help to protect the newborn against infection. Taken as a supplement, colostrum can boost the immune system and help the body to burn fat and build lean muscle. It may also accelerate the healing of injuries, increase vitality and stamina, and have an anti-aging effect. Supplemental colostrum usually contains bovine (cow) colostrum. Good sources include New Life Colostrum from Symbiotics (both original and high-Ig formulas) and Colostrum Specific from Jarrow Formulas.

Corn Germ

Corn germ is made by a process that isolates the embryo of the corn plant, which contains the most usable nutrients. Corn germ has a longer shelf life than wheat germ and is higher in some nutrients, especially zinc. Corn germ contains ten times the amount of zinc found in wheat germ. You can use corn germ to bread chicken or fish. It is also good when added to cereals and used as a topping.

Creatine

Creatine (creatine monohydrate) is a compound produced by metabolic processes in the body. When muscles are in use, the compound adenosine triphosphate (ATP) is broken down into two other compounds—adenosine diphosphate (ADP) and inorganic phosphate. This process produces the body's cellular energy, which, among other things, powers the muscles. Each such burst of energy is very fleeting. However, with the addition of creatine, ADP can be transformed back to ATP, the source of cellular energy. Taken as a supplement, creatine can increase both endurance and strength, making possible extended workout time. Longer workouts in turn can result in increased lean muscle mass.

Creatine is particularly popular with athletes. The use of creatine for muscle-depleting illnesses and the natural wasting of muscles that comes with age is also being studied. Creatine should be used in combination with a balanced, nutritionally complete diet. You should not take it with fruit juices, as this combination results in the production of creatinine, which is difficult for the kidneys to process. Never exceed the recommended dose.

Dehydroepiandrosterone (DHEA)

Dehydroepiandrosterone (DHEA) is a hormone that is produced primarily by the adrenal glands and is found naturally in the human body. It is an important base from which other key substances, including the hormones testosterone, progesterone, and corticosterone, can be derived, either directly or indirectly. The amount of DHEA produced by the body declines with age, particularly after age forty. Research indicates that taking DHEA supplements may help to prevent cancer, arterial disease, multiple sclerosis, and Alzheimer's disease; may be beneficial in the treatment of lupus and osteoporosis; may enhance the activity of the immune system; and may help to improve memory.

However, caution should be exercised when taking this supplement. Some physicians believe that taking high doses of DHEA suppresses the body's natural ability to synthesize this hormone. Further, laboratory studies have shown that high doses can lead to liver damage. If you take supplemental DHEA, it is important also to take supplements of the antioxidant vitamins C and E and the antioxidant mineral selenium to prevent oxidative damage to the liver. Possible side effects of taking DHEA include excess growth of facial hair in women. This can often be avoided by starting with a dose of 10 milligrams daily. 7-Keto DHEA is a derivative of DHEA that is not converted into estrogen or testosterone, which is good for women concerned about breast cancer and for men concerned about prostate cancer. 7-Keto DHEA is a good alternative to DHEA and has the same benefits.

Desiccated Liver

Desiccated liver is concentrated dried liver that is put into powdered or tablet form. This form of liver contains vitamins A, D, and C; the B-complex vitamins; and the minerals calcium, copper, phosphorus, and iron. Desiccated liver is good for people with anemia, and aids in building healthy red blood cells. It is known to increase energy, aid in liver disorders, and help relieve stress in the body. Use only a product made from liver derived from beef that is raised organically.

Dimethylglycine (DMG)

Dimethylglycine (DMG) is a derivative of glycine, the simplest of the amino acids. It acts as a building block for many important substances, including the amino acid methionine, choline, a number of important hormones and neurotransmitters, and DNA.

Low levels of DMG are present in meats, seeds, and grains. It is a safe, nontoxic food substance that does not build up in the body. No deficiency symptoms are associated with a lack of DMG in the diet, but taking supplemental DMG can have a wide range of beneficial effects, including helping the body maintain high energy levels and boosting mental acuity. DMG has been found to enhance the immune system and to reduce elevated blood cholesterol and triglyceride levels. It improves oxygen utilization by the body, helps to normalize blood pressure and blood glucose levels, and improves the functioning of many important organs. It may also be useful for controlling epileptic seizures. Some people have used DMG as a substitute for pangamic acid, a supplement that is no longer available in the United States but that is widely used in Russia to treat heart disease, liver disease, alcohol and drug addiction, and other problems. DMG is thought to increase pangamic acid levels in the body. Aangamik DMG from FoodScience Laboratories is a good source of supplemental DMG.

161

Dimethylaminoethanol (DMAE)

Dimethylaminoethanol (DMAE) is similar to choline, a chemical involved in the processes of learning and memory. It has been known to be beneficial for people with autism, memory deficiency, and dementia. It is best not to take it on a daily basis, but to reserve it for days when you need to increase alertness and focus. DMAE can have a slight mood- and vision-enhancing effect in some people. Lifespan 2000 from Country Life is a good source of supplemental DMAE.

Dimethylsulfoxide (DMSO)

Dimethylsulfoxide (DMSO) is a byproduct of wood processing for papermaking. It is a somewhat oily liquid that looks like mineral oil and has a slightly garlicky odor. Because it is an excellent solvent, it is widely used as a degreaser, paint thinner, and antifreeze. However, it also has remarkable therapeutic properties, especially for the healing of injuries. Applying DMSO on sprained ankles, pulled muscles, dislocated joints, and even at the site of simple fractures can virtually eliminate the pain. It also promotes immune-system activity.

DMSO is absorbed through the skin and enters the bloodstream by osmosis through capillary walls. It is then distributed through the circulatory system and ultimately is excreted through the urine. It has been used successfully in the treatment of brain and spinal cord damage, arthritis, Down syndrome, sciatica and other back problems, keloids, acne, burns, musculoskeletal problems, sports injuries, cancer, sinusitis, headaches, skin ulcers, herpes, and cataracts.

Essential Fatty Acids (EFAs)

Fatty acids are the basic building blocks of which fats and oils are composed. Contrary to popular myth, the body does need fat. It must be the right kind, however.

The fatty acids that are necessary for health and that cannot be made by the body are called *essential fatty acids* (EFAs). They are occasionally also referred to as *vitamin F* or *polyunsaturates*. EFAs must be supplied through the diet.

Essential fatty acids have desirable effects on many disorders. They improve the skin and hair, reduce blood pressure, aid in the prevention of arthritis, lower cholesterol and triglyceride levels, and reduce the risk of blood clot formation. They are beneficial for candidiasis, cardiovascular disease, eczema, and psoriasis. Found in high concentrations in the brain, EFAs aid in the transmission of nerve impulses and are needed for the normal development and functioning of the brain. A deficiency of essential fatty acids can lead to an impaired ability to learn and recall information.

Every living cell in the body needs essential fatty acids. They are essential for rebuilding and producing new cells. Essential fatty acids are also used by the body for the production of prostaglandins, hormonelike substances that act as chemical messengers and regulators of various body processes.

There are two basic categories of essential fatty acids, designated *omega-3* and *omega-6*, based on their chemical structures. Omega-3 EFAs, including alpha-linolenic and eicosapentaenoic acid (EPA), are found in fresh deepwater fish, fish oil, and certain vegetable oils, among them canola oil, flaxseed oil, and walnut oil. Omega-6 EFAs, which include linoleic and gamma-linolenic acids, are found primarily in raw nuts, seeds, and legumes, and in unsaturated vegetable oils, such as borage oil, grape seed oil, primrose oil, sesame oil, and soybean oil. In order to supply essential fatty acids, these oils must be consumed in pure liquid or supplement form and must not be subjected to heat, either in processing or cooking. Heat destroys essential fatty acids. Worse, it results in the creation of dangerous free radicals (*see* chapter six—ANTIOXIDANTS). If oils are hydrogenated (processed to make the oil more solid, as is commonly done in the production of margarine), the linoleic acid is converted into trans-fatty acids, which are not beneficial to the body.

The daily requirement for essential fatty acids is satisfied by an amount equivalent to 10 to 20 percent of total caloric intake. The most essential of the essential fatty acids is linoleic acid.

A number of sources of essential fatty acids are recommended in this book, among them fish oils, flaxseeds and flaxseed oil, grape seed oil, and primrose oil.

EMU OIL Emu oil is an excellent source of linoleic acid, linolenic acid, and oleic acid, which have anti-inflammatory properties. It can be used topically for the relief of rashes, hemorrhoids, poison ivy, insect bites, arthritis, joint aches, muscle strains, and it has been known to stop the pain of burns. It can also be used as a facial moisturizer to reduce wrinkles and lines. Emu Oil and Emu Plus from Emu Country, Inc. are good sources of Emu oil.

FISH OIL Fish oil is a good source of omega-3 essential fatty acids. Salmon, mackerel, menhaden, herring, and sardines are good sources of fish oil because they have a higher fat content and provide more omega-3 factors than other fishes. For instance, 4 ounces of salmon contains up to 3,600 milligrams of omega-3 fatty acids, while 4 ounces of cod (a low-fat fish) contains only 300 milligrams.

Carlson Laboratories markets a good Norwegian salmon oil that we recommend. Cod liver oil from Norway is the most commonly used fish oil and is more mild tasting than other varieties. Author Dale Alexander claims it is excellent for arthritis. He has marketed an oil containing 13,800 international units of vitamin A and 1,380 international units of vitamin D per tablespoon. However, we do not recommend that you rely on cod liver oil as a source of the essential fatty acids. You would have to overdose on vitamins A and D to obtain the amount of fatty acids you need.

People with diabetes should not take fish oil supplements because of the high fat content, but they should consume fish for its essential fatty acids.

FLAXSEEDS AND FLAXSEED OIL Flaxseeds are rich in omega-3 essential fatty acids, magnesium, potassium, and fiber. They are also a good source of the B vitamins, protein, and zinc. They are low in saturated fats and calories, and contain no cholesterol. The nutty taste of ground flaxseeds is pleasant, and they can be mixed with water or any fruit or vegetable juice. They can also be added to salads, soups, yogurt, cereals, baked goods, or fresh juices. You can grind these tiny seeds in a coffee grinder.

If you prefer not to eat the seeds, you can use flaxseed oil as an alternative. Like the seeds from which it is extracted, organic cold-pressed flaxseed oil is rich in essential fatty acids. Several studies have shown that it can reduce the pain, inflammation, and swelling of arthritis. It has been found to lower blood cholesterol and triglyceride levels, and to help reduce the hardening effects of cholesterol on cell membranes.

GRAPE SEED OIL Of the many natural sources of essential fatty acids, grape seed oil is among the highest in linoleic acid and among the lowest in saturated fats. It contains no cholesterol and no sodium. It has a light, nutty taste that brings out the flavor in many foods. Unlike most other oils, it can be heated to temperatures as high as 485°F without producing dangerous and possibly carcinogenic free radicals. These features make it good for use in cooking. Buy only grape seed oil that is cold-pressed and contains no preservatives, such as Salute Santé Grapeseed Oil from Lifestar International.

PRIMROSE OIL Primrose oil (also known as evening primrose oil) contains 9 to 10 percent gamma-linolenic acid (GLA). This fatty acid is known to help prevent hardening of the arteries, heart disease, premenstrual syndrome, multiple sclerosis, and high blood pressure. It relieves pain and inflammation; enhances the release of sex hormones, including estrogen and testosterone; aids in lowering cholesterol levels; and is beneficial for cirrhosis of the liver.

165

Many women have found that primrose oil supplements relieve unpleasant menopausal symptoms such as hot flashes. Because it promotes the production of estrogen, women suffering from breast cancer that is diagnosed as estrogen-receptor positive (estrogen-related) should avoid or limit their intake of primrose oil. Black currant seed oil is a good substitute.

COMBINATION EFA SUPPLEMENTS A product called Ultimate Oil from Nature's Secret contains a blend of cold-pressed organic oils that offers a good balance of both omega-3 and omega-6 fatty acids. A purely vegetable-based product, Ultimate Oil contains extra-virgin flaxseed oil, black currant seed oil, pumpkin seed oil, lecithin, and safflower oil. We also recommend Kyolic-EPA from Wakunaga of America, a blend of aged garlic extract and fish oil derived from northern Pacific sardines, and Cardiovascular Research's Essential Fatty Acid Complex.

Evening Primrose Oil

See Primrose Oil *under* Essential Fatty Acids above.

Fiber

Found in many foods, fiber helps to lower blood cholesterol levels and stabilize blood sugar levels. It helps prevent colon cancer, constipation, hemorrhoids, obesity, and many other disorders. Fiber is also good for removing certain toxic metals from the body. Because the refining process has removed much of the natural fiber from our foods, the typical American diet is lacking in fiber.

There are seven basic classifications of fiber: bran, cellulose, gum, hemicellulose, lignin, mucilages, and pectin. Each form has its own function. It is best to rotate among several different supplemental fiber sources. Start with small amounts and gradually increase your intake until your stools are the proper consistency. Also, be aware that while today's average diet is lacking in fiber, consuming excessive amounts may decrease the absorption of zinc, iron, and calcium. Always take supplemental fiber separately from other medications or supplements. Otherwise, it can lessen their strength and effectiveness.

In addition to using a fiber supplement, you should make sure to get fiber through your diet. Make sure your diet contains these high-fiber foods: whole-grain cereals and flours, brown rice, agaragar, all kinds of bran, most fresh fruit, dried prunes, nuts, seeds (especially flaxseeds), beans, lentils, peas, and fresh raw vegetables. Eat several of these foods daily. When eating organic produce, leave the skin on apples and potatoes. Coat chicken in corn bran or oats for baking. Add extra bran to cereals and breads. Unsalted, unbuttered popcorn is also excellent for added fiber.

BRAN, GUMS, AND MUCILAGES Both gums and mucilages help to regulate blood glucose levels, aid in lowering cholesterol, and help in the removal of toxins. They are found in oatmeal, oat bran, sesame seeds, and dried beans.

One of the following should be part of your daily dietary plan:

- *Fennel seed.* Fennel is an herb that is helpful for digestive purposes. The seeds of this plant help to rid the intestinal tract of mucus and aid in relieving flatulence.
- *Glucomannan.* Derived from the tuber of the amorphophallis plant, it picks up and removes fat from the colon wall. This substance is good for diabetes and obesity because it helps to get rid of fat. It has been recognized for normalizing blood sugar and is good for people with hypoglycemia. Glucomannan expands to sixty times its own weight, thereby helping to curb the appetite. Taking 2 to 3 capsules with a large glass of water thirty minutes before meals is helpful for reducing allergic reactions and some symptoms associated with high and low blood sugar disorders. Always be sure to drink a large glass of water when taking glucomannan in capsule or pill form, as capsules can lodge in the throat and expand there, causing breathing problems. Glucomannan is tasteless and odorless, and can be added to foods to help normalize blood sugar.
- *Guar gum.* Extracted from the seeds of the guar plant, guar gum is good for the treatment of diabetes and for curbing the appetite. It also has the ability to reduce the levels of cholesterol, triglycerides, and low-density lipoproteins in the blood, and binds with toxic substances and carries them out of the body. Guar gum tablets must be chewed thoroughly or sucked gradually, not swallowed whole, and should be taken with lots of water, because guar gum has a tendency to ball up in the throat when mixed with saliva. It should not be used by individuals who have difficulty swallowing or who have had gastrointestinal surgery. Some persons with colon disorders may have trouble using guar gum.
- *Oat bran and rice bran.* Bran is the broken coat of the seed of cereal grain that has been separated from the flour or meal by sifting or bolting. It helps to lower cholesterol.
- *Psyllium seed.* Psyllium is a grain grown in India that is utilized for its fiber content. A good intestinal cleanser and stool softener, it is one of the most popular fibers used. It thickens very quickly when mixed with liquid, and must be consumed im-

mediately. Some doctors recommend Metamucil, which contains psyllium hydrophilic mucilloid, as a laxative and fiber supplement. However, we prefer less processing and all-natural products.

CELLULOSE Cellulose is an indigestible carbohydrate found in the outer layer of vegetables and fruits. It is good for hemorrhoids, varicose veins, colitis, and constipation, and for the removal of cancer-causing substances from the colon wall. It is found in apples, beets, Brazil nuts, broccoli, carrots, celery, green beans, lima beans, pears, peas, and whole grains.

HEMICELLULOSE Hemicellulose is an indigestible complex carbohydrate that absorbs water. It is good for promoting weight loss, relieving constipation, preventing colon cancer, and controlling carcinogens in the intestinal tract. Hemicellulose is found in apples, bananas, beans, beets, cabbage, corn, green leafy vegetables, pears, peppers, and whole grain cereals.

LIGNIN This form of fiber is good for lowering cholesterol levels. It helps to prevent the formation of gallstones by binding with bile acids and removing cholesterol before stones can form. It is beneficial for persons with diabetes or colon cancer. Lignin is found in Brazil nuts, carrots, green beans, peaches, peas, potatoes, strawberries, tomatoes, and whole grains.

PECTIN Because it slows the absorption of food after meals, pectin is good for people with diabetes. It also removes unwanted metals and toxins, reduces the side effects of radiation therapy, helps lower cholesterol, and reduces the risk of heart disease and gallstones. Pectin is found in apples, bananas, beets, cabbage, carrots, citrus fruits, dried peas, and okra.

COMBINATION FIBER SUPPLEMENTS There are many products available that combine two or more different types of fiber, or that combine fiber with other ingredients. Three products of this kind that we recommend are:

- Aerobic Bulk Cleanse (ABC) from Aerobic Life Industries. This product is an excellent source of fiber. It contains blond psyllium seed husks and the herbs licorice and hibiscus. This therapeutic drink aids in healing and cleansing the colon. It is excellent for diarrhea and constipation. Add it to a combination of one-half aloe vera juice and one-half fruit juice. Be sure to take this mixture on an empty stomach, first thing in the morning. Stir it well and drink it down quickly, before it thickens. Related products, also from Aerobic Life Industries, include 10-Day Colon Cleanse and 45-Day Cleanse for Colon, Blood, and Lymph.

- Aerobic Colon Care from Aerobic Life Industries. This formula contains psyllium and oat bran, and provides approximately 3 grams of soluble fiber and 4 grams of insoluble fiber per serving.
- A.M/P.M. Ultimate Cleanse from Nature's Secret. This formula combines gums with cellulose, hemicellulose, pectin, and lignin, plus herbs that support and cleanse the blood and internal organs. It is a two-part system for stimulating and detoxifying the entire body.

Fish Oil

169

See under Essential Fatty Acids in this section.

5-Hydroxy L-Tryptophan (5-HTP)

5-HTP is a substance that is created naturally in the body from the amino acid tryptophan, and that in turn is used by the body to produce serotonin, an important neurotransmitter. Supplemental 5-HTP is derived from the seeds of the griffonia plant (*Griffonia simplicifolia*), which is native to western Africa. It can be used to aid in weight loss, insomnia, and depression. In a sense, 5-HTP can be seen as a substitute for supplemental L-tryptophan, which is no longer available in the United States (*see* chapter five—AMINO ACIDS). 5-HTP should be used together with a high-carbohydrate food or liquid such as orange juice, and as part of a comprehensive nutritional program. It may not benefit everyone who takes it. If you regularly take large doses of 5-HTP (more than 300 milligrams daily), you should undergo blood testing for eosinophil (a type of white blood cell) levels every three months. HTP.Calm from Natural Balance is a good source of 5-HTP. You should avoid this supplement if you are taking antidepressants.

Flaxseeds and Flaxseed Oil

See under Essential Fatty Acids in this section.

Garlic

Garlic is one of the most valuable foods on this planet. It has been used since Biblical times and is mentioned in the literature of the ancient Hebrews, Greeks, Babylonians, Romans, and Egyptians. The builders of the pyramids supposedly ate garlic daily for endurance and strength.

Garlic lowers blood pressure through the actions of one of its components, methyl allyl trisulfide, which dilates blood vessels. It thins the blood by inhibiting platelet aggregation, which reduces the risk of blood clots and aids in preventing heart attacks. It also lowers serum cholesterol levels and aids in digestion. Garlic is useful for many diseases and illnesses, including cancer. It is a potent immune system stimulant and a natural antibiotic. It should be consumed daily. It can be eaten fresh, taken in supplement form, or used to prepare garlic oil.

Garlic contains an amino acid derivative, alliin. When garlic is consumed, the enzyme alliinase, which converts alliin to allicin, is released. Allicin has an antibiotic effect; it exerts an antibacterial effect estimated to be equivalent to 1 percent of that of penicillin. Because of its antibiotic properties, garlic was used to treat wounds and infections and to prevent gangrene during World War I.

Garlic is also effective against fungal infections, including athlete's foot, systemic candidiasis, and yeast vaginitis, and there is some evidence that it may also destroy certain viruses, such as those associated with fever blisters, genital herpes, a form of the common cold, smallpox, and a type of influenza.

Garlic oil is good for the heart and colon, and is effective in the treatment of arthritis, candidiasis, and circulation problems. To make garlic oil, add peeled whole garlic cloves to a quart of olive or canola oil. Experiment to find the number of cloves that gives the degree of flavor you like. Be sure to wash your hands thoroughly and rinse the garlic after peeling and before placing it in the oil. The peel may contain mold and bacteria that can contaminate the oil. Keep this oil refrigerated. This mixture will keep for up to a month before you need to replace it with fresh oil. Garlic oil can be used for sautéing, in salad dressings, and in a variety of other ways. If you find the odor too strong after you eat garlic, chew some sprigs of parsley or mint, or caraway or fennel seeds.

An alternative to fresh garlic is Kyolic from Wakunaga of America. Kyolic is an odorless, "sociable" garlic product, and is available in tablet, capsule, and oil extract forms.

Ginkgo Biloba

The ornamental tree *Ginkgo biloba* originated in China thousands of years ago, and now grows in temperate climates throughout the world. The extract of its fan-shaped leaves is one of the world's most popular herbal products. It has been reported in scientific journals to enhance blood circulation and to increase the supply of oxygen to the heart, brain, and all bodily parts. This makes it useful for improving memory and relieving muscle pains. It also acts as an antioxidant, has anti-aging effects, reduces blood pressure, inhibits blood clotting, and is helpful for tinnitus, vertigo, hearing loss, impotence, and Raynaud's disease. Ginkgo biloba is widely known as the "smart herb" of our time. It has even been shown to slow the early progression of Alzheimer's disease in some individuals.

Ginseng

Ginseng is used throughout the Far East as a general tonic to combat weakness and give extra energy. There are a number of different types of ginseng: *Eleutherococcus senticosus* (Siberian ginseng), *Panax quinquefolium* (American ginseng), *Panax ginseng* (Chinese or Korean ginseng), and *Panax japonicum* (Japanese ginseng). *Panax ginseng* is the most widely used species.

Early Native Americans were familiar with ginseng. They called it *gisens* and used it for stomach and bronchial disorders, asthma, and neck pain. Russian scientists claim that the ginseng root stimulates both physical and mental activity, improves endocrine gland function, and has a positive effect on the sex glands. Ginseng is beneficial for fatigue because it spares glycogen (the form of glucose stored in the liver and muscle cells) by increasing the use of fatty acids as an energy source. It is used to enhance athletic performance, to rejuvenate, to increase longevity, and to detoxify and normalize the entire system.

In lower doses, ginseng seems to raise blood pressure, while higher amounts appear to reduce blood pressure. Research suggests that high doses of ginseng may be helpful for inflammatory diseases such as rheumatoid arthritis, without the side effects of steroids, and may also protect against the harmful effects of radiation. Ginseng is beneficial for people with diabetes because it decreases the level of the hormone cortisol in the blood (cortisol interferes with the function of insulin). However, people with hypoglycemia should avoid using large amounts of ginseng.

The root is sold in many forms: as a whole root or root pieces, which are either untreated or blanched; as a powder or powdered extract; as a liquid extract or concentrate; in granules for instant tea; as a tincture; in an oil base; and in tablets and capsules. These products should not contain sugar or added color, and should be pure ginseng. Many supplement manufacturers add ginseng to combination products, but these often contain such low amounts that they may not be effective. Wakunaga of America distributes several high-quality Korean and Siberian ginseng products.

We advise following the Russian approach to using ginseng: Take it for fifteen to twenty days, followed by a rest period of two weeks. Avoid long-term usage of high doses.

Glucomannan

See under Fiber in this section.

Glucosamine

This is one of a number of substances classified as an *amino sugar.* Unlike other forms of sugar in the body, amino sugars are components of carbohydrates that are incorporated into the structure of body tissues, rather than being used as a source of energy. Glucosamine is thus involved in the formation of the nails, tendons, skin, eyes, bones, ligaments, and heart valves. It also plays a role in the mucous secretions of the digestive, respiratory, and urinary tracts.

Glucosamine is made in the body from the simple carbohydrate glucose and the amino acid glutamine. It is found in high concentrations in joint structures. It is also available as a supplement, in the form of glucosamine sulfate, which helps to combat both the causes and symptoms of osteoarthritis. Glucosamine has been proven in over 300 studies and 20 clinical trials to actually build joint cartilage. It can also slightly reduce the destruction of cartilage and depression caused by taking nonsteroidal anti-inflammatory drugs (NSAIDs), which are commonly prescribed for people with arthritis. Glucosamine may be taken in conjunction with chondroitin sulfate for an even greater effect on osteoarthritis (*see* Chondroitin Sulfate in this section).

In addition to having benefits for people with osteoarthritis, supplemental glucosamine can be helpful for asthma, bursitis, candidiasis, food allergies, osteoporosis, respiratory allergies, tendinitis, vaginitis, and various skin problems. GS-500 from Enzymatic Therapy is a good source of glucosamine. GlucosaMend from Source Naturals, Glucosamine Plus from FoodScience Laboratories, and Glucosamine Sulfate Complex from PhytoPharmica are other recommended products. A related compound is N-acetylglucosamine (NAG), available as N-A-G from Source Naturals.

Grape Seed Oil
See under Essential Fatty Acids in this section.

"Green Drinks"
"Green drinks" are natural food formulas made from plants that are good detoxifiers and blood cleansers, as well as sources of chlorophyll, minerals, enzymes, and other important nutrients. Generally, they are sold in powdered form to be mixed just before use.

Many different companies market green drink formulas. The following are some recommended products:

- Barley Green from AIM International. This product contains a combination of barley juice and kelp.
- Earthsource Greens & More from Solgar. This formula combines four organically grown grasses (alfalfa, barley, kamut, and wheat), Hawaiian blue-green spirulina, and Chinese chlorella with three potent immune-stimulating mushrooms (maitake, reishi, and shiitake), plus powdered broccoli, carrots, and red beets, which supply phytonutrients. Its fruit flavor comes from fresh fruit powders.
- Green Magma from Green Foods Corporation. Green Magma is a pure, natural juice of young barley leaves that are organically grown in Japan and are pesticide-free. Brown rice is added to supply vitamins B_1 (thiamine) and B_3 (niacin), and linoleic acid. Green Magma contains thousands of enzymes, which play an important role in the metabolism of the body (*see* chapter seven—ENZYMES), plus a high concentration of superoxide dismutase (SOD). The powdered product may be added to juice or quality water.
- Kyo-Green from Wakunaga of America. This is a combination of barley, wheatgrass, kelp, and the green algae chlorella. The barley and wheatgrass are organically grown. It is a highly concentrated natural source of chlorophyll, amino acids, vitamins and minerals, carotene, and enzymes. Chlorella is a rich natural source of vitamin A, and kelp supplies iodine and other valuable minerals. (*See* Chlorella and Kelp in this section.)
- ProGreens from NutriCology. ProGreens includes organic alfalfa, barley, oat, and wheatgrass juice powders; natural fiber; wheat sprouts; blue-green algae; sea algae; fructooligosaccharides (FOS); lecithin; standardized bioflavonoid extracts; royal jelly and bee pollen; beet and spinach extracts; acerola juice powder; natural vitamin E; and the herbs astragalus, echinacea, licorice, Siberian ginseng, and suma.

Green Papaya

Green (unripe) papaya is an excellent source of vitamins, minerals, and enzymes. Ounce for ounce, it contains more vitamin A than carrots and more vitamin C than oranges, as well as abundant B vitamins and vitamin E. The complex of enzymes it contains helps to digest proteins, carbohydrates, and fats.

Green papaya can be eaten fresh or taken in supplement form. Papain is the most abundant, most active enzyme in both the fresh fruit and the powdered supplement form. Papain possesses very powerful digestive action. A good source of green papaya is Mature Green Papaya Powder from Papaya John's. Papaya John's makes a variety of papaya bars, including Papaya Ginger & NONI Turmeric Milk Thistle & Flax, which is a papaya bar that is very beneficial for the internal organs (especially the liver), Papaya Almond, and Papaya Macadamia Nut. The same company also produces a Papaya Honey concentrate that can be used as a replacement for sugar, honey, or syrup, or as a jam.

175

Guar Gum

See under Fiber in this section.

Hemicellulose

See under Fiber in this section.

Honey

Bees produce honey by mixing nectar, which is a sweet substance secreted by flowers, with bee enzymes. Honey is made up of 35 percent protein and contains half of all the amino acids, and is a highly concentrated source of many essential nutrients, including large amounts of carbohydrates (sugars), some minerals, B-complex vitamins, and vitamins C, D, and E.

Honey is used to promote energy and healing. It is a natural antiseptic and makes a good salve for burns and wounds. Honey is also used for sweetening other foods and beverages. It varies somewhat in color and taste depending on the origin of the flower and nectar, but in general it is approximately twice as sweet as sugar, so not as much is needed for sweetening purposes. People who have diabetes or hypoglycemia should be careful when consuming honey and its by-products. These substances affect blood sugar levels in the same way that refined sugars do. Tupelo honey contains more fructose than other types of honey and it is absorbed at a slower rate, so some people with hypoglycemia can use this type sparingly without ill effects.

Buy only unfiltered, unheated, unprocessed honey, and *never* give honey to an infant under one year of age. In its natural form, honey can contain spores of the bacteria that cause botulism. This poses no problem for adults and older children, but in infants, the spores can colonize the digestive tract and produce the deadly botulin toxin there. Honey is safe for babies after age one.

Inosine

Inosine occurs naturally in the human body. It is involved in the rebuilding of adenosine triphosphate (ATP; see page 150), and stimulates the production of a compound designated 2,3-disphosphoglycerate (2,3-DPG), which is needed in the transportation of oxygen to muscle cells for the production of energy. Weight and endurance trainers have found supplemental inosine to be beneficial; it is believed to increase muscle development and blood circulation. It also enhances immune function.

If you have kidney problems or gout, you should not take inosine because it contains nitrogen and can increase the production of uric acid. For best results, use the dosage recommended by the manufacturer for your body size, and take it forty-five to sixty minutes prior to exercising.

Inositol Hexaphosphate (IP$_6$)

Inositol hexaphosphate (IP$_6$, also known as phytic acid) is a compound consisting of the B vitamin inositol plus six phosphate groups. Found naturally in many foods, including wheat, rice, and legumes, it is a powerful antioxidant that has many positive effects on the body. Laboratory studies suggest it may fight cancer, prevent and treat heart disease, prevent kidney stones and liver disease, and also reduce cholesterol levels and prevent the inappropriate formation of blood clots, a major cause of heart attacks. IP_6 inhibits the activity of free radicals in the body, which slows the type of abnormal cell division associated with cancer and tumor growth. It works best very early in the development of malignant tumors, before the malignancy can even be recognized by the immune system. The cells are then normalized and begin to grow in the usual manner again.

IP_6 contains a substance designated beta-1,3-D-glucan, which helps to maintain a strong immune system in people undergoing chemotherapy and radiation. IP_6 protects the heart by preventing the formation of blood clots in blood vessels and reducing the levels of cholesterol and triglycerides (fats) in the bloodstream. It protects the liver by preventing fatty deposits from accumulating there. Studies have shown that a diet high in IP_6 is associated with a lower incidence of cancer of the breast, colon, and prostate.

Significant amounts of IP_6 are found in foods such as beans, brown rice, whole-kernel corn, sesame seeds, wheat bran, cornbread, grape juice, raisins, and mulberries. It can also be taken in supplement form. Some studies have shown that IP_6 may interfere with the body's absorption of minerals, so supplements should not be taken within one hour of meals. IP_6 from Jarrow Formulas and Cell Forté with IP-6 from Enzymatic Therapy are recommended sources of IP_6.

177

Kelp

Kelp is a type of seaweed that can be eaten raw, but it is usually dried, granulated, or ground into powder. It is also available in a liquid form that can be added to drinking water. Granulated or powdered kelp can be used as a condiment and for flavoring, as a salt substitute. If you find the taste unappealing, you can purchase it in tablet form.

Kelp is a rich source of vitamins, especially the B vitamins, as well as of many valuable minerals and trace elements. It is reported to be very beneficial to brain tissue, the membranes surrounding the brain, the sensory nerves, and the spinal cord, as well as the nails and blood vessels. It has been used in the treatment of thyroid problems because of its iodine content, and is useful for other conditions as varied as hair loss, obesity, and ulcers. It protects against the effects of radiation and softens stools. Kelp is recommended as a daily dietary supplement, especially for people with mineral deficiencies.

Kombucha Tea

The kombucha, or Manchurian "mushroom," has reputedly been used in Asian countries and in Russia for centuries. The "mushroom" itself is not eaten. Rather, a tea is made by fermenting the "mushroom" for about a week in a mixture of water, sugar, and green or black tea, with apple cider vinegar or a bit of previously made tea added. Kept in this mixture, the "mushroom" reproduces, and the "daughter mushrooms" can then be used to produce more tea.

Although commonly referred to as a mushroom, the kombucha is actually a combination of a number of different elements, including lichen, bacteria, and yeast. Kombucha tea contains a variety of different nutrients and other health-promoting substances. It is a natural energy booster and detoxifier that may also help slow or reverse the aging process and fight such serious diseases as AIDS, cancer, and multiple sclerosis.

Because of the way in which it has traditionally been propagated (one at a time, by individual users), kombucha may be difficult to find. Many people who have them received a daughter "mushroom" as a gift from a friend, although there are some herbal companies that sell both the "mushrooms" and the bottled tea commercially.

Lactobacillus Acidophilus

Lactobacillus acidophilus is a type of "friendly" bacteria that assists in the digestion of proteins, a process in which lactic acid, hydrogen peroxide, enzymes, B vitamins, and antibiotic substances that inhibit pathogenic organisms are produced. Acidophilus has antifungal properties, helps to reduce blood cholesterol levels, aids digestion, and enhances the absorption of nutrients.

The flora in the healthy colon should consist of at least 85 percent lactobacilli and 15 percent coliform bacteria. However, the typical colon bacteria count today is the reverse. This can result in gas, bloating, intestinal and systemic toxicity, constipation, and malabsorption of nutrients, and is conducive to an overgrowth of candida. Taking an acidophilus supplement helps to combat all of these problems by returning the intestinal flora to a healthier balance. In addition, acidophilus may help to detoxify harmful substances.

There are many good acidophilus supplements available. Acidophilus products come in tablet, capsule, and powdered forms. We recommend using the powdered form. Natren markets quality products that contain very high numbers of organisms. Nondairy formulas are best for people who are allergic to dairy products, and they work well against candida. Probiata from Wakunaga of America is a milk-free product that remains stable at high temperatures. Other good nondairy acidophilus supplements include Primadophilus from Nature's Way, Neo-Flora from New Chapter, and Flora from DaVinci Labs. In general, we believe it is not advisable to buy a product containing a combination of different strains of lactobacilli, as one organism may be antagonistic to another. A single-strain product with a count of at least 1 billion organisms per gram is often better than a combination.

Acidophilus can die at high temperatures. Whatever product you choose, keep it in a cool, dry place—refrigerate but do not freeze it. Take acidophilus on an empty stomach in the morning and one hour before each meal. If you are taking antibiotics, do not take the antibiotics and acidophilus simultaneously.

Lactoferrin

Lactoferrin is a protein that occurs naturally in human bile, tears, mucus, saliva, and milk. Because it binds with free iron in the body, it plays an important role in regulating iron levels (and, in turn, growth) and aids in preventing and fighting infection by depriving disease-causing organisms of the iron they need to grow and multiply. It also plays a role in the functioning of lymphocytes, a type of white blood cell important for immunity. Taken in sup-

179

plement form, it may boost immune function and help in combating both infectious and inflammatory conditions. It may also benefit intestinal health.

Lecithin

Lecithin is a type of lipid that is needed by every living cell in the human body. Cell membranes, which regulate the passage of nutrients into and out of the cells, are largely composed of lecithin. The protective sheaths surrounding the brain are composed of lecithin, and the muscles and nerve cells also contain this essential fatty substance. Lecithin consists mostly of the B vitamin choline, and also contains linoleic acid and inositol. Although lecithin is a lipid, it is partly soluble in water and thus acts as an emulsifying agent. This is why many processed foods contain lecithin.

This nutrient helps to prevent arteriosclerosis, protects against cardiovascular disease, improves brain function, and aids in the absorption of thiamine by the liver and vitamin A by the intestine. It is also known to promote energy and is needed to help repair damage to the liver caused by alcoholism. Lecithin enables fats, such as cholesterol and other lipids, to be dispersed in water and removed from the body. The vital organs and arteries are thus protected from fatty buildup.

Lecithin would be a wise addition to anyone's diet. It is especially valuable for older adults. Anyone who is taking niacin for high serum cholesterol and triglycerides should also include lecithin in his or her program. Two tablespoons of lecithin granules can be sprinkled on cereals and soups or added to juices or breads. Lecithin also comes in capsule form. Taking one 1,200-milligram capsule before each meal helps in the digestion of fats and the absorption of fat-soluble vitamins.

Most lecithin is derived from soybeans, but recently egg lecithin has become popular. This type of lecithin is extracted from the yolks of fresh eggs. Egg lecithin may hold promise for those suffering from AIDS, herpes, chronic fatigue syndrome, and immune disorders associated with aging. Studies have shown that it works better for people with these disorders than soy lecithin does. Other sources of lecithin include brewer's yeast, grains, legumes, fish, and wheat germ.

Lignin

See under Fiber in this section.

Maitake

Maitake (*Grifola frondosa*) is a mushroom that has a long history of use in traditional Chinese and Japanese herbology and cooking. It grows wild in Japan, as well as in some wooded areas in eastern North America. Because maitake is difficult to cultivate, however, only relatively recently have the mushrooms become widely available.

Maitake is considered an adaptogen, which means that it helps the body adapt to stress and normalizes bodily fuctions. Its healing properties are thought to be related to its high content of a polysaccharide called beta-1,6-glucan, which is considered very powerful. In laboratory studies, this substance has been shown to prevent carcinogenesis, inhibit the growth of cancerous tumors, kill HIV, and enhance the activity of key immune cells known as T-helper cells or CD4 cells. Maitake may also be useful for diabetes, chronic fatigue syndrome, chronic hepatitis, obesity, and high blood pressure.

Research suggests that maitake is better absorbed than other mushrooms, such as shiitake, and it is almost as effective when taken orally as it is when taken intravenously. Maitake can be eaten in food or taken as a supplement. Buy organically grown dried mushrooms (when using them in cooking, soak them in water or broth for half an hour first), or purchase maitake in capsule, extract, or tea form. Some of the capsule supplements contain a small amount of vitamin C, which enhances the effectiveness of the active ingredient in maitake by aiding in its absorption.

Melatonin

The hormone melatonin is naturally produced by the pineal gland, a cone-shaped structure in the brain. The body's pattern of melatonin production is similar to that of the other "anti-aging"

181

MAINTAINING YOUR MELATONIN LEVEL NATURALLY

As darkness falls at the end of each day, melatonin production rises. In the morning, when daylight hits the retina, neural impulses cause production of the hormone to slow. Clearly, light and darkness are the primary factors that set the rhythms of melatonin production. However, they are not the only factors involved. In fact, it has been found that a variety of regular daily routines can strengthen the rhythm of melatonin production. Here are a few simple ways in which you can help your body maintain high levels of this important hormone:

- Eat regular meals. The rhythm of melatonin production is strengthened by regular daily routines. Keep your mealtimes as regular as possible to keep your body in sync with the rhythms of the day.

- Keep your diet light at night. When melatonin production begins after nightfall, the digestive process is slowed. Thus, any heavy foods eaten close to bedtime may lead to digestive problems, which can make it difficult to sleep. To get the sleep you need, eat small, light meals in the late evening.

- Avoid stimulants. Stimulants like coffee, tea, and caffeine-containing medications and soft drinks can interfere with melatonin production by interfering with your sleep. As much as possible, eliminate these stimulants from your diet and lifestyle.

- Avoid exercising late at night. Vigorous activity delays melatonin secretion. If you exercise in the morning, you will reinforce healthful sleeping habits that lead to regular melatonin production. For best results, do your morning exercise outdoors, in the morning light.

hormones, human growth hormone (HGH) and dehydroepiandrosterone (DHEA). Throughout early life, melatonin is produced in abundance. Shortly before puberty, though, the production of melatonin begins to drop, and then continues to decline steadily as we age.

Research has demonstrated that melatonin may have several

profound long-term effects on the body. As one of the most powerful antioxidants ever discovered—with a greater range of effectiveness than vitamin C, vitamin E, or beta-carotene—melatonin helps prevent harmful oxidation reactions from occurring. In this way, melatonin may prevent the changes that lead to hypertension and heart attack, and may reduce the risk of certain kinds of cancer. Indeed, research has indicated that many age-related problems are caused by declining levels of melatonin, which leave the body less able to prevent and repair oxidative damage. Melatonin also has been found to stimulate the immune system; have a major role in the production of estrogen, testosterone, and possibly other hormones, helping to prevent cancers involving the reproductive system; and slow the growth of existing malignancies. Recent studies suggest that if melatonin is taken in the mornings, tumor growth may be stimulated, but if it is taken in the evenings, tumor growth tends to be slowed. In addition, as melatonin is secreted cyclically, in response to the fall of darkness at the end of each day, the hormone helps our bodies keep in sync with the rhythms of day and night. Thus, melatonin helps regulate sleep.

183

Research on melatonin continues, and with it, knowledge is increasing about the functions of melatonin in the body and the effects of melatonin supplementation. Both human research studies and anecdotal evidence indicate that melatonin supplements can be an effective and side-effect-free sleep aid both for adults suffering from insomnia and for children with autism, epilepsy, Down syndrome, cerebral palsy, and other problems that can cause sleep disorders. Animal and other laboratory research indicates that melatonin supplementation may help prevent age-related disorders, and perhaps extend life. Melatonin can be taken to ease PMS symptoms; stimulate the immune system; prevent memory loss, arteriosclerosis, and stroke; and treat cancer and Alzheimer's disease.

Although no toxic levels of melatonin have been found, some researchers feel that certain people probably should not use this supplement until further information is available. Included in this category are pregnant and nursing women; people with severe allergies or autoimmune diseases; people with immune system cancers, such as lymphoma and leukemia; and healthy children, who already produce sufficient amounts of the hormone. Since high doses of melatonin have been found to act as a contraceptive, women who wish to become pregnant also might want to avoid taking this supplement.

Melatonin should be taken two hours or less before bedtime. This schedule is designed to release the added hormone at the same time that natural production peaks. A sustained-release form is best if you frequently awaken after several hours' sleep; a sublingual form is best if you are very ill or suffer from malabsorption. When you awaken after melatonin-assisted sleep, you should feel refreshed—not tired or groggy. If you do experience grogginess, you should reduce the dosage. (To learn how you can maintain or increase your melatonin levels through daily routines, *see* Maintaining Your Melatonin Level Naturally, on page 182.)

Methylsulfonylmethane (MSM)

Methylsulfonylmethane (MSM, also known as dimethylsulfone) is a naturally occurring organic sulfur compound found in plant and animal tissues that is essential for optimum health. It is a derivative of dimethysulfoxide (DMSO), which has remarkable therapeutic properties, especially for the healing of injuries. It can also help to detoxify the body on a cellular level. MSM helps to nourish the hair, skin, and nails; relieve pain and inflammation; reduce allergy problems; and promote gastrointestinal health. It has also been found to aid immune function, and there have been reports of benefits to patients with heartburn, arthritis, lung problems, migraines, and muscle pain.

MSM is present naturally in foods such as fresh fish, meat, plants, fruit, and milk. However, it can be eliminated by even moderate processing, including drying or heating. Since most North Americans today eat considerable amounts of processed food, MSM is normally either not present at all or present only in very small amounts in the typical diet. Most people therefore would probably benefit from supplementation.

Research suggests that we require a constant supply of MSM for optimum good health, as sulfur is one of the essential minerals. Commonly recommended dosage levels are about 2,000 milligrams (2 grams) per day taken in divided doses, with the morning and evening meals, but it is best to start out at 1,000 milligrams (1 gram) per day to avoid a too-rapid rate of detoxification. Benefits usually become evident in two to twenty-one days, and can be enhanced by vitamin C supplementation. MSM from Aerobic Life Industries and OptiMSM from Cardinal Nutrition are good sources of this nutrient. Natrol produces a good MSM supplement as well.

Mucilage

See under Fiber in this section.

Nicotinamide Adenine Dinucleotide (NADH)

NADH is a form of vitamin B_3 (niacin) that is essential for the production of various neurotransmitters and cellular energy. NADH, which is also known as coenzyme 1, also acts as an antioxidant (*see* chapter six—ANTIOXIDANTS).

185

As we age, natural levels of NADH decline, which can lead to reduced levels of both energy and significant brain chemicals. Taking supplemental NADH can result in improvements in the biochemistry of energy production, especially in the brain and nervous systems. NADH shows promise as a therapy for Parkinson's disease because it results in an increase in brain levels of the neurotransmitter dopamine, which is deficient in people with this disorder. People with Alzheimer's disease may be helped by this supplement as well. Some people suffering from chronic fatigue syndrome (CFS) have shown significant improvement with NADH therapy. ENADA (NADH) from Kal Dietary Supplements is a good source of NADH.

Oat Bran

See under Fiber in this section.

Octacosanol

Octacosanol is a naturally derived wheat germ oil concentrate. (Although it would be possible to extract octacosanol from whole wheat, 10 pounds of wheat would be needed to obtain just 1,000 micrograms of octacosanol.) Wheat germ has long been known for its many benefits. Today, extracts of wheat germ weighing only 2 milligrams offer remarkable benefits as well.

Octacosanol has been clinically proven to increase oxygen utilization during exercise and improve glycogen stores in muscle tissue. As a result, it increases physical endurance, improves reaction time, reduces high-altitude stress, and aids in tissue oxygenation. This substance can greatly benefit those who experience muscle pain after exercise or have a lowered endurance level. It is good for muscular dystrophies and other neuromuscular disorders as well. It also reduces blood cholesterol levels.

186

Olive Leaf Extract

Olive leaf extract is an herbal supplement that has been shown to be effective against virtually all the viruses and bacteria on which it has been tested. Laboratory studies suggest that olive leaf extract interferes with viral infection becoming established and/or spreading, either by rendering viruses incapable of infecting cells or by preventing them from reproducing. It has been shown to help protect against infection by such viruses as human immunodeficiency virus (HIV), herpesviruses, and influenza viruses. It is useful for such disorders as pneumonia, sore throat, sinusitis, and skin diseases such as chronic infections and rashes, as well as for fungal and bacterial infections. Olivir from DaVinci Laboratories is a good source of olive leaf extract that has been tested in clinical trials.

Pectin

See under Fiber in this section.

Perilla

Perilla (*Perilla frutescens*) is an Asian plant that is a member of the mint family. It has been prescribed by Asian herbalists for the relief of cough and lung ailments, and for certain types of food poisoning, as well as to prevent the flu and restore energy balance. It may aid in increasing learning ability and is also used as a culinary herb.

Perilla comes in several forms, including seed oil. This is an unsaturated oil that contains linolenic, linoleic, and oleic acids. Perilla oil is available in capsule form. Studies suggest that it may be an effective and safe source of essential omega-3 fatty acids.

Phosphatidyl Choline

Phosphatidyl choline (PC) is a component of lecithin (*see* Lecithin in this section). Taken as a supplement, it helps to break down fats and can be helpful in preventing atherosclerosis (hardening of the arteries due to fatty plaques in the blood vessels), heart disease, gallstones, and liver problems. It is has also shown substantial benefits for people with neurological disorders, memory loss, and depression. PC is known to be safe and effective; however, people with manic-depressive disorder should not take large amounts.

Phosphatidyl Serine

Phosphatidyl serine (PS) is a substance classified as a phospholipid (a phosphorus-containing lipid) that is needed by every cell in the body, and is especially abundant in nerve cells. PS is the most important of the phospholipids and is crucial for the maintenance of healthy cell membranes. Although the brain normally produces enough PS, production dwindles as we age, which can result in deficiency.

Supplemental PS, which is compounded from soybean oil, has been found to reduce symptoms of depression and Alzheimer's disease, and to enhance memory and learning abilities. Some people have experienced nausea as a result of taking PS; however, taking it with food can help to avoid this. No danger has been reported with long-term use of this supplement. Its safety for pregnant women has not been determined.

Pregnenolone

Pregnenolone is a steroid hormone that the body normally manufactures from cholesterol, and that in turn can be metabolized into a variety of other vital hormones, including DHEA, progesterone, testosterone, and estrogen. The body's own pregnenolone levels decline with age, and many scientists believe that pregnenolone supplements may treat symptoms commonly associated with aging. Other benefits of using pregnenolone may include improved brain function that manifests itself as enhanced mood, memory, and thinking. Pregnenolone has also been known to lower cholesterol levels and alleviate the symptoms of conditions as varied as Alzheimer's disease, lupus, multiple sclerosis, premenstrual syndrome (PMS), rheumatoid arthritis, scleroderma, seizures, psoriasis, prostate disorders, stress, trauma, injuries, sleep disorders, and chronic fatigue syndrome. It also increases the effectiveness of hormone replacement therapy and the immune system.

It is important to use caution in taking supplemental pregnenolone. It has not yet been studied as thoroughly as other hormones that are available over the counter; consequently, its full effects on the body are not yet conclusively known. Until more information is available, it may be best to use the lowest effective dosage and to seek the supervision of a knowledgeable health care provider. Reported side effects of pregnenolone include headache, insomnia, irritability, anxiety, mood swings, irregularities of heartbeat, acne, growth of facial hair, and loss of scalp hair.

Primrose Oil

See under Essential Fatty Acids in this section.

Probiotics

Probiotics are beneficial bacteria normally present in the digestive tract. They are vital for proper digestion and also perform a number of other useful functions, such as preventing the overgrowth of yeast and other pathogens, and synthesizing vitamin K. The probiotics most often used as supplements are acidophilus and bifidobacteria (*see Lactobacillus acidophilus* and/or *Bifidobacterium bifidum* in this section). Cultured, or fermented, foods also contain various types and amounts of beneficial bacteria. These foods include buttermilk, cheese, kefir, miso, sauerkraut, tempeh, umeboshi, and yogurt.

Progesterone Cream

Progesterone is a hormone that is produced primarily by the ovaries and also by the adrenal glands. It works in partnership with estrogen to regulate menstrual cycles and is important for the maintenance of pregnancy. In addition to its role in the female reproductive system, it has a number of other important effects: it stimulates the activity of bone-building cells called osteoblasts; exerts an antidepressant and calming effect in the brain; helps to regulate blood sugar levels; and plays a role in maintaining the myelin sheaths that protect nerve cells. It can be used by the body to produce other hormones, including DHEA, estrogen, testosterone, and cortisol, as needed. A deficiency of progesterone, on the other hand, can exacerbate symptoms of premenstrual syndrome (PMS) and menopausal discomforts, and may increase the risk of osteoporosis. Progesterone deficiency becomes increasingly common in women as they approach menopause, and can start as early as age thirty-five. Symptoms can include night sweats, hot flashes, depression, and premenstrual discomfort.

Supplemental progesterone is available in cream form. The hormone is absorbed through the skin after the cream is applied, and it passes directly into the bloodstream for transport to sites where progesterone is needed. Natural Woman Essential Body Cream from Products of Nature and Endocreme 900 Extra Strength from Wuliton Labs are recommended products.

Propolis

See Bee Propolis in this section.

Psyllium Seed

See under Fiber in this section.

189

Red Yeast Rice

Red yeast rice is a food product created by fermenting rice with a strain of red yeast (*Monascus purpureus,* Went yeast). It is also sometimes referred to as Monascus rice or, in Chinese, *Hung-chu* or *Hong-Qu.* It has long been used in China and Japan as a food and as a remedy for digestive ailments and poor circulation. More recently, red yeast rice extract, taken in supplement form, has been found both to reduce overall blood cholesterol levels and to improve the ratio of HDL ("good cholesterol") to LDL ("bad cholesterol"). A study conducted by the University of California—Los Angeles School of Medicine found that people who took red yeast rice and maintained a low-fat diet reduced their overall cholesterol levels by an average of 40 points over a period of twelve weeks. The extract contains a number of cholesterol-lowering compounds known as *statins.* One of these is lovastatin, a substance also sold as a prescription drug under the brand name Mevacor. Lovastatin acts to lower cholesterol by inhibiting the action of an enzyme designated HMG-CoA reductase, which in turn limits the rate at which the body produces cholesterol. Studies have shown statins to lower cholesterol levels and reduce the risk of heart attack. Unlike prescription products, red yeast rice extract has shown no serious adverse side effects in clinical trials.

Reishi

See Shiitake and Reishi in this section.

Rice Bran

See under Fiber in this section.

Royal Jelly

Royal jelly is a thick, milky substance that is secreted from the pharyngeal glands of a special group of young nurse bees between their sixth and twelfth days of life. When honey and pollen are combined and refined within the young nurse bee, royal jelly is naturally created. This substance contains all of the B-complex vitamins, including a high concentration of pantothenic acid (vitamin B_5) and vitamin B_6 (pyridoxine), and is the only natural source of pure acetylcholine. Royal jelly also contains minerals, enzymes, hormones, eighteen amino acids, antibacterial and antibiotic components, and vitamins A, C, D, and E. It is useful for bronchial asthma, liver disease, pancreatitis, insomnia, stomach ulcers, kidney disease, bone fractures, and skin disorders, and it strengthens the immune system.

This product must be combined with honey to preserve its potency. Royal jelly spoils easily. Keep it refrigerated and make sure it is tightly sealed when purchased.

S-adenosylmethionine (SAMe)

S-adenosylmethionine (SAMe) is a derivative of the amino acid methionine that is formed in the body when methionine combines with adenosine triphosphate (ATP), the major source of cellular energy. Taken as a supplement, SAMe has a variety of positive effects: it is an effective antidepressant; it is beneficial for disorders of the joints and connective tissue, including arthritis and fibromyalgia; it promotes the health of the liver; and it may lower levels of homocysteine, a dangerous amino acid that is associated with cardiovascular disease. It may also help to slow the aging process. SAMe works closely with folic acid, choline, and vitamins B_6 and B_{12}. It is one of a class of substances called *methyl donors*. As the name implies, methyl donors are compounds that "donate" units called methyl groups, which contain hydrogen and carbon atoms, to other substances. This process is called *methylation*, and it is one way in which the body protects itself from damage on the cellular level. Among other things, methyl donors help to protect against such serious disorders as cancer, heart disease, neurological disorders, and many age-related problems, and facilitate the manufacture of DNA and brain neurotransmitters. Taking supplemental SAMe may also increase natural levels of glutathione, an antioxidant; phosphatidyl choline, which aids in the metabolism of fats; and the hormone melatonin. A small number of people have experienced minor nausea and gastrointestinal disturbances as a result of taking high doses, but otherwise no notable side effects have been reported. Although SAMe is considered very safe, anyone with manic-depressive disorder (bipolar mood disorder) should consult a physician before taking this supplement. SAMe should always be taken on an empty stomach.

Sea Cucumber

Sea cucumbers, also known as *bêche de mer* and *trepang,* are not actually cucumbers, but are marine animals related to starfishes and sea urchins. They have been used in China for thousands of years as a treatment for arthritis. Modern research has confirmed they are beneficial for musculoskeletal inflammatory diseases, especially rheumatoid arthritis, osteoarthritis, and ankylosing spondylitis, a rheumatic disease that affects the spine.

Researchers believe that sea cucumbers improve the balance of prostaglandins, which regulate the inflammatory process. They also contain substances known as chondroitins, which are often lacking in people with arthritis and connective tissue disorders (*see* Chondroitin Sulfate in this section). In addition, sea cucumbers provide vitamins A, B_1 (thiamine), B_2 (riboflavin), and B_3 (niacin), and C, as well as the minerals calcium, iron, magnesium, and zinc. Sea Cucumber from Futurebiotics is a good source of this supplement.

Sea Mussel

The green-lipped mussel (*Perna canaliculus*) is a species of edible shellfish. They contain numerous amino acids, the building blocks of body proteins, in addition to enzymes and essential trace elements. The minerals they contain are present in a balance similar to that in blood plasma, and these minerals are naturally chelated by the amino acids, making for better assimilation into the body.

Sea mussel aids in the functioning of the cardiovascular system, the lymphatic system, the endocrine system, the eyes, connective tissues, and mucous membranes. They help to reduce inflammation and relieve the pain and stiffness of arthritis. They also promote the healing of wounds and burns.

Shark Cartilage

The tough, elastic material that makes up the skeleton of the shark is dried and pulverized (finely powdered) to make this food supplement. Shark cartilage contains a number of active components, the most important of which is a type of protein that acts as an angiogenesis inhibitor—that is, it acts to suppress the development of new blood vessels. This makes it valuable in fighting a number of disorders. Many cancerous tumors, for instance, are able to grow only because they induce the body to develop new networks of blood vessels to supply them with nutrients. Shark cartilage suppresses this process, so that tumors are deprived of their source of nourishment and, often, begin to shrink. There are also certain eye disorders, such as diabetic retinopathy and macular degeneration, that are characterized by the growth of new blood vessels within the eye; because they grow in inappropriate places, the presence of these blood vessels can lead to blindness. Such diseases also may respond well to shark cartilage. Other conditions for which shark cartilage is useful include arthritis, psoriasis, and regional enteritis (inflammation of the lining of the bowels). In addition to angiogenesis-inhibiting protein, shark cartilage contains calcium (approximately 16 percent) and phosphorus (approximately 8 percent), which are absorbed as nutrients, and mucopolysaccharides that act to stimulate the immune system.

193

Shark cartilage is available in powder and capsule forms. Exercise caution when buying shark cartilage, as the purity and correct processing of the product are vital to its effectiveness. Not all shark cartilage products contain only 100-percent pure shark cartilage, so read labels carefully. Pure shark cartilage is white in color. If you find the odor and/or taste of pure shark cartilage to be stronger than you can tolerate, look for a product called BeneFin, which has significantly less fishy taste and smell than most other products. BeneFin is a trademarked name for naturally processed shark cartilage manufactured by Lane Labs–USA and marketed by various companies under license. If you are taking large quantities of shark cartilage, it may be wise to increase your supplementation of certain minerals, especially magnesium and potassium, to maintain a proper mineral balance in the body. Shark cartilage should *not* be taken by pregnant women or children, or by persons who have recently undergone surgery or suffered a heart attack.

Shiitake and Reishi

Shiitake and reishi are Japanese mushrooms with a delicate texture, strong stems, and well-defined undersides. They are attractive and have impressive health-promoting properties.

Shiitake (*Lentinus edodes*) contain a polysaccharide, lentinan, that strengthens the immune system by increasing T cell function. Shiitake mushrooms contain eighteen amino acids, seven of which are essential amino acids. They are rich in B vitamins, especially vitamins B_1 (thiamine), B_2 (riboflavin), and B_3 (niacin). When sundried, they contain high amounts of vitamin D. Their effectiveness in treating cancer has been reported in a joint study by the Medical Department of Koibe University and Nippon Kinoko Institute in Japan. These mushrooms are considered delicacies and are entirely edible.

Reishi (*Ganoderma lucidum*) have been popular for at least 2,000 years in the Far East. They were rated number one on ancient Chinese lists of superior medicines, and were believed to give eternal youth and longevity.

Today, both shiitake and reishi mushrooms are used to treat a variety of disorders and to promote vitality. They are used to prevent high blood pressure and heart disease, to control and lower cholesterol, to build resistance to disease, and to treat fatigue and viral infections. They are also known to have anti-tumor properties valuable in treating cancer.

The mushrooms are available fresh or dried for use in foods (soak dried mushrooms in warm water or broth for thirty minutes before using), as well as in supplements in capsule, pill, and extract form.

Spirulina

Spirulina is a microalgae that thrives in hot, sunny climates and in alkaline waters around the world, and produces twenty times as much protein as soybeans growing on an equal-sized area of land. It contains concentrations of nutrients unlike any other single grain, herb, or plant. Among its valuable components are gamma-linolenic acid (GLA), linoleic and arachidonic acids, vitamin B_{12} (needed, especially by vegetarians, for healthy red blood cells), iron, a high level of protein (60 to 70 percent), essential amino acids, the nucleic acids RNA and DNA, chlorophyll, and phyco-cyanin, a blue pigment that is found only in blue-green algae and that has increased the survival rate of mice with liver cancer in laboratory experiments.

Spirulina is a naturally digestible food that aids in protecting the immune system, in cholesterol reduction, and in mineral absorption. Because it supplies nutrients needed to help cleanse and heal, while also curbing the appetite, it is beneficial for people who are fasting. A person with hypoglycemia may benefit from using this food supplement between meals because its high protein content helps stabilize blood sugar levels.

Torula Yeast

See Yeast in this section.

Wheat Germ

Wheat germ is the embryo of the wheat berry. It is a good source of vitamin E; most of the B vitamins; the minerals calcium, magnesium, and phosphorus; and several trace elements.

One problem with wheat germ is that it spoils easily. If you purchase wheat germ separately from the flour, make sure the product is fresh. It should be either vacuum packed or refrigerated, with a packing date or a label stating the date by which the product should be used. Toasted wheat germ has a longer shelf life, but the raw product is better because it is unprocessed. Wheat germ oil capsules are also available.

Wheatgrass

Wheatgrass is a rich nutritional food that was popularized by Dr. Ann Wigmore, an educator and founder of the Hippocrates Health

Institute in Boston. Wheatgrass contains a great variety of vitamins, minerals, and trace elements. According to Dr. Wigmore, 1 pound of fresh wheatgrass is equal in nutritional value to nearly 25 pounds of the choicest vegetables.

Dr. Wigmore reported that wheatgrass therapy, along with "living foods," helped to eliminate cancerous growths and helped many other disorders, including mental health problems. The molecular structure of chlorophyll resembles that of hemoglobin, the oxygen-carrying protein of red blood cells, and this may be the reason for the effectiveness of wheatgrass. The key difference between the two is that the metallic atom in the middle of each molecule of human hemoglobin is iron, while the metallic atom at the center of a molecule of chlorophyll is magnesium. In experiments on anemic animals, blood counts returned to normal after four to five days of receiving chlorophyll.

Whey Protein

Whey is a normal byproduct of cheesemaking; it is the liquid that is left when the solids in milk come together and are pressed into solid form. Whey protein is produced by filtering and purifying whey, then removing the water to produce a powder that, while high in quality protein, is free of fat and lactose (milk sugar).

This supplement helps to build lean body mass by increasing the body's production of muscle protein. For this reason, it is popular among athletes and bodybuilders, and also helps to protect against muscle-wasting in people with such diseases as AIDS and cancer. In addition to its effect on muscles, it appears to inhibit the proliferation of cancer cells, protect against free radical damage, and enhance immune function. Some recommended whey protein supplements include Biochem Whey Pro 290 from Country Life, Molkosan Whey of Life from Bioforce A.G., ProFlora Whey from Healing Arts Association, and Whey to Go from Solgar.

Yeast

Yeast are single-celled organisms that can multiply at extremely rapid rates, doubling in number in two hours. Yeast is rich in many basic nutrients, such as the B vitamins (except for vitamin B$_{12}$), sixteen amino acids, and at least fourteen different minerals. The protein content of yeast is responsible for 52 percent of its weight. Yeast is also high in phosphorus.

There are various media on which yeast may be grown. Brewer's yeast, also known as nutritional yeast, is grown on hops, a bitter herb that is also used as an ingredient in beer. Torula yeast is grown on blackstrap molasses or wood pulp. A liquid yeast product from Switzerland called Bio-Strath, distributed by Bioforce of America, is derived from herbs, honey, and malt. It is a natural product that we highly recommend.

Live baker's yeast should be avoided. Live yeast cells actually deplete the body of B vitamins and other nutrients. In nutritional yeast, these live cells are destroyed, leaving the beneficial nutrients behind.

Yeast may be consumed in juice or water, and is a good energy booster between meals. It can also be added to the diet to aid in treating certain disorders. It helps in sugar metabolism and is good for eczema, heart disorders, gout, nervousness, and fatigue. By enhancing the immune system, yeast is useful for people undergoing radiation therapy or chemotherapy for cancer. Yeast also seems to increase mental and physical efficiency. Dr. William Crook, author of *The Yeast Connection* (Vintage Books, 1986), states that if a person with candida-related health problems is not specifically allergic to yeast, it is all right for him or her to take a food supplement containing yeast. However, we suggest avoiding yeast products if candidiasis is suspected. Because yeast contains significant amounts of phosphorus, people suffering from osteoporosis should avoid yeast products. Those who do take yeast should be sure to take extra calcium as well.

Specialty Supplements

In addition to the substances discussed above, there are many natural food supplements designed for specific circumstances. There are too many of these products for us to discuss all of them here, but several that we feel are to be highly recommended are the following:

197

- Allergy Relief formulas from bioAllers. These are eight homeopathic formulas designed to relieve allergies by combining homeopathic remedies with specific allergens to help strengthen resistance to those allergens. Formulas include Animal Hair/Dander; Grain/Dairy; Grass Pollen; Mold/Yeast/Dust; Pollen/Hayfever; Sinus & Allergy Nasal Spray; and Tree Pollen.

- Arthogesic from Enzymatic Therapy. This is a topical gel designed to provide temporary relief from minor muscle aches, joint pain associated with arthritis, backache, bruises, strains, and sprains. The active ingredient is capsaicin, a compound derived from cayenne pepper (capsicum).

- Artichoke from Nature's Plus Herbal Actives. This supplement contains artichoke extract standardized to a minimum of 2.5 to 5 percent caffeylquinic acids, and also contains sesquiterpene lactones and the highly active flavonoids scolymoside, inulin, and taraxasterol. It is designed to support the liver and circulatory system.

- Betatene from NatureWorks. This is a dietary supplement of mixed carotenoids, including alpha- and beta-carotene, lutein, lycopene, zeaxanthin, and cryptoxanthin. It is intended to help maintain a healthy and strong immune system.

- Body Language Essential Green Foods from Oxyfresh USA. This is a combination that includes alfalfa, Atlantic kelp, kale, spinach, spirulina, bladderwrack, dulse, barley grass, chlorella, dunaliella, and wheatgrass, plus the enzymes maltase, amylase, protease, lipase, cellulase, and pectinase, to provide a green food concentrate rich in beta-carotene, chlorophyll, and trace minerals.

- Bone Maximizer from Metabolic Response Modifiers. This is a combination supplement that contains microcrystalline hydroxyapatite concentrate (MCHC). MCHC is a source of bone proteins and highly absorbable calcium. Other ingredients include glucosamine, pregnenolone, vitamin D, magnesium, methylsulfonylmethane (MSM, a source of bioavailable sulfur), and other nutrients vital for bone health.

- Bone Support with Ostivone from Twinlab. This is a combination supplement designed to help maintain healthy bones. Ingredients include ipriflavone, calcium, vitamin D, magnesium, boron, and purified soy phytoestrogen extracts.

- BotanImmune from Bodyonics. This is a hypoallergenic dietary supplement designed to boost the immune system. Ingredients include thymus fractions, olive leaf extract, raspberry-ellagic acid, soy isoflavones, beta-1,3-glucan, and indole-3-carbinol, a compound found in broccoli, cabbage, and other cruciferous vegetables that has shown promise as an immune-boosting and anticancer substance.

- Breast Health from NaturalMax. This supplement contains the soy isoflavone genistein, black currant blend, freeze-dried broccoli, indole-3-carbinol, the herbs gotu kola and saw palmetto, and lycopene.

- CamoCare cream from Abkit. This product contains chamomile and other active ingredients. It relieves pain associated with a variety of ailments involving the muscles and joints, such as backache, arthritis, and pain from inflamed joints.

- Cardiaforce from Bioforce AG. This hawthorn berry extract promotes healthy cardiovascular function, circulation, and heart-muscle strength. It is a liquid supplement that is meant to be added to water and taken three times a day, before meals. It has no known interactions with other medications, and should be taken over a period of several months, with periodic short interruptions.

- Chromium Picolinate from Superior Source. This is a sublingual form of chromium picolinate that is particularly good for children, older adults, and people with malabsorption problems. Chromium picolinate promotes the burning of fat by the body, increases lean muscle mass, and helps to speed up the metabolism (*see* chapter three—MINERALS).

- Cold, flu and allergy season formulas from ZAND. This is a line of products designed to support health through the various allergy seasons of the year. Individual formulas include Insure Herbal, an echinacea and goldenseal formula; Decongest Herbal, a natural decongestant formula; HerbalMist throat spray; and Allergy Season, which contains bromelain, nettle extract, quercetin, and vitamin B_5 (pantothenic acid). These formulas can be used individually or on a rotating basis.

- Diamond Mind from Diamond-Herpanacine Associates. This product combines a number of herbal extracts and nutrients, including ginkgo biloba, gotu kola, ginseng, garlic, phosphatidyl serine, and phosphatidyl choline, in a supplement intended to support and improve memory, concentration, and mental energy and alertness.

- Diamond Trim from Diamond-Herpanacine Associates. This is a supplement program intended to promote weight loss by helping control appetite, reduce food cravings, increase the burning of calories, and reduce the absorption of fats. It also contains minerals to replenish those often lost through dieting. Ingredients include fiber, digestive enzymes, the herbs St. John's wort and griffonia, the minerals calcium and potassium, and a trace mineral complex.

- Earth's Bounty NONI from Matrix Health Products. Noni (*Morinda citrifolia*) is a small tree that grows in Hawaii and other tropical regions. The fruit of this plant has a long history of use for a wide variety of problems, including joint problems, pain, inflammation, digestive problems, and cardiovascular disorders. Its active compounds include phytochemicals, designated anthraquinones, enzymes, and alkaloids.

- Echinaforce from Bioforce. This is a liquid echinacea supplement that promotes natural disease resistance during the winter season and helps to maintain a healthy immune system.

- EstroGentle from Bodyonics. This is an herbal supplement designed to help support women's health during and after menopause. Ingredients include phytoestrogen-containing botanicals such as black cohosh and soy isoflavones, as well as chaste tree berry (*Vitex agnus-castus*), dong quai, licorice root, red clover leaf extract, and wild yam root.

- Fibroplex from Metagenics. This supplement contains vitamins B_1 (thiamine) and B_6 (pyridoxine), magnesium, manganese, and malic acid. It is designed to provide nutritional support for the nerves and muscles.

- GastroSoothe from Enzymatic Therapy. GastroSoothe is a natural antacid that contains calcium carbonate, deglycyrrhizinated licorice extract (DGL), and the amino acid glycine for the relief of indigestion and heartburn.
- Herbal Mood Boost from Country Life. This supplement contains a complex of herbs and nutrients known for their positive effects on mood and anxiety, including St. John's wort, 5-hydroxytryptophan (5-HTP), Siberian ginseng, kava kava, and passionflower.
- Hyper-C Serum from Jason Natural Cosmetics. This is an oil-based moisturizing formula that contains vitamin C, an antioxidant, to protect the skin from free radical damage. It also reduces the appearance of existing fine lines and wrinkles, evens out skin tones, and makes the skin softer and smoother in texture.
- HyperiCalm from Enzymatic Therapy. This supplement contains St. John's wort extract standardized to provide 0.3 percent hypericin. It is designed to support mental and nervous system function (*see* St. John's Wort under Herbs and Their Uses in chapter nine—HERBS).
- Instant Enerjetz from Superior Source. This is a convenient, easy-to-take form of vitamin B_{12} that is placed on or under the tongue (not swallowed). Vitamin B_{12} is needed to prevent anemia and maintain a healthy nervous system, and it boosts energy and combats fatigue (*see* chapter two—VITAMINS).
- Jerusalem artichoke tablets. Jerusalem artichoke whole tuber flour (JAF) tablets are a good source of fructooligosaccharides (FOS), which support the growth of healthy intestinal flora.
- Kava-30 from Enzymatic Therapy. This supplement provides kava kava extract standardized to contain 30 percent kavalactones. It is designed to soothe and support the central nervous system (*see* Kava Kava under Herbs and Their Uses in chapter nine—HERBS).
- Kolorex from Forest Herbs. Kolorex is an herbal antifungal product that contains extract of the native New Zealand shrub *Pseudowintera colorata* and anise seed oil. Taken in capsule form, it aids in balancing the bacteria in the gastrointestinal tract,

preventing an overgrowth of candida. There is also a topical cream form that can be applied directly to surface fungal infections, including athlete's foot, jock itch, and nail infections. The manufacturer recommends that the two forms of this product be used in combination for best results.

- Kyolic Neuro Logic from Wakunaga of America. This supplement contains aged garlic extract, ginkgo biloba extract, lecithin, acetyl-L-carnitine, and phosphatidyl serine in a formula designed to improve memory and mental activity.

- Maxi-Calm from Prevail Corporation. Maxi-Calm is a dietary supplement containing kava kava, valerian, passion flower, skullcap, and wild lettuce, each of which has traditionally been used to support the nervous system.

- Micellized Multiple Vitamin and Minerals from Earth Science, Inc. This is a liquid multivitamin and mineral supplement that is easily absorbed and utilized by the body.

- Miracle 2000 from Century Systems, Inc. is a combination supplement that contains twenty-seven vitamins and minerals, eighteen herbs, eight amino acids, and numerous ionic trace minerals.

- Nature's Answer FOR KIDS. This is a line of herbal extracts designed for children. They are made using alcohol, like standard extracts, but the alcohol is then removed and replaced with glycerin, which is a preservative and a natural sweetener. Formulas include Bubble B-Gone, a combination colic remedy containing catnip, chamomile, fennel, and lemon balm; KID Catnip; KID Chamomile; E-KID-nacea, an echinacea extract; E-KID-nacea Plus, which contains echinacea and goldenseal; Ginger KID; KID B-Well Tonic, an immune-system tonic containing astragalus, burdock, and dandelion; NAT-Choo: a cold and flu remedy containing a blend of boneset, catnip, echinacea, eyebright, and peppermint; and Tummie Tonic, an indigestion remedy including angelica, chamomile, fennel, ginger, meadowsweet, and slippery elm.

- Osteo-Max from Metabolic Response Modifiers. This supplement contains ipriflavone, an isoflavone similar to those found in soybeans and soy products, and microcrystalline hydroxyapatite concentrate (MCHC; *see under* Bone Maximizer, above). It is designed to support both bone metabolism and the maintenance of bone density.

- Phytodolor from Enzymatic Therapy. This liquid supplement contains extracts of common ash, aspen, and goldenrod; the key compounds include salicylic acid derivatives, phenolic acid, flavonoids, and triterpene saponins. Phytodolor is intended to support muscle and joint function without causing stomach irritation, as many other products used for the relief of arthritis and similar disorders do.

- PreNatal Care from Natrol. This is a combination supplement designed for pregnant women and nursing mothers. Ingredients include essential vitamins, minerals, and antioxidants, among them the B vitamin folic acid and the omega-3 essential fatty acid docosahexaenoic acid (DHA), that are necessary for a healthy pregnancy and healthy prenatal development.

- Quick Cleanse Program from ZAND. This is a program utilizing three separate supplements: Cleansing Fiber formula, a fiber supplement containing psyllium seed and husk, plus bentonite and kaolin; Cleansing Laxative formula, with cascara sagrada (an herbal stimulant laxative) and kaolin; and Thistle Cleanse formula, a milk thistle supplement. This combination of formulas is designed to cleanse the intestinal tract, eliminate toxins, and support liver function.

- Remifemin and Remifemin Plus from Enzymatic Therapy. Remifemin is a standardized extract of black cohosh that has been used in Europe for over forty years for the treatment of menopausal symptoms. Remifemin Plus also contains standardized St. John's wort extract, which has been found to combat depression and improve the sense of emotional well-being (*see* Black Cohosh and St. John's Wort under Herbs and Their Uses in chapter nine—HERBS). These supplements do not affect hormone levels.

- Smart Longevity from E'Ola Products. This liquid supplement is designed to bolster brain function. It contains nutrients to enhance brain function and antioxidants to protect against free radical damage. Ingredients include vitamin C, ginseng extract, schizandra extract, dimethylaminoethanol (DMAE), choline, and vitamin E.

- Soy-Licious from Country Life. This dietary supplement is a high-protein soy-based drink mix with added genistein and daidzein (soy isoflavones), essential vitamins and minerals, antioxidants, and adaptogenic herbs (adaptogens are herbs that help the body adapt to and cope with the effects of stress).

- Sub-Adrene from American Biologics. This is a highly concentrated whole adrenal-cortical extract of bovine origin. Designed for sublingual administration, it has a peppermint taste and supplies a balance of natural steroids.

- Super Green Tea Extract from Prolongevity. This supplement contains 95 percent green tea extract standardized to 35 percent epigallocatechin gallate. It is available in two forms, regular and decaffeinated. Studies have indicated that green tea can help to protect against stroke and heart attack, and may even inhibit the growth of cancer cells (*see* Green Tea under Herbs and Their Uses in chapter nine—HERBS).

- Ultra High Performance Dietary Supplement from Excel. This supplement contains a blend of energizing herbs and is designed to provide the body with a quick boost of energy without caffeine.

- Ultra Juice Green from Nature's Plus. This is a supplement based on marine algae and containing a total of twenty different green foods in tablet form. It contains a wide range of vitamins, minerals, and phytonutrients.

- VitaSerum from ABRA Therapeutic Skin Care. This is a skin-care product designed to protect against free radicals, stimulate cell renewal, and reduce the visible signs of aging. It contains vitamin C from acerola berries; herbal extracts of elder flower, green tea, grape seed, and horsetail; citrus and cranberry bioflavonoids; hyaluronic acid; zinc sulfate; and essential oils of lavender, rose geranium, and sweet lavender.

- Vita Synergy for Men from The Synergy Company. This is a combination nutritional supplement that contains a balanced blend of all major vitamins and minerals, trace elements, and a variety of herbal extracts used to support men's health.

- Wellness Formula from Source Naturals. This supplement is designed to support optimal health in cold weather. Its ingredients include vitamins A and C, beta-carotene, and bioflavonoids; the immune-boosting mineral zinc; bee propolis; and the herbs angelica, astragalus, boneset, cayenne, echinacea, garlic, goldenseal, hawthorn berry, horehound, mullein, pau d'arco, and Siberian ginseng.

NINE

Herbs

The medicinal benefits of herbs have been known for centuries. Records of Native American, Roman, Egyptian, Persian, and Hebrew medical practices show that herbs were used extensively to cure practically every known illness. Many herbs contain powerful ingredients that, if used correctly, can help heal the body. The pharmaceutical industry was originally based upon the ability to isolate these ingredients and make them available in a purer form. Herbalists, however, contend that nature provides other ingredients in the same herbs to balance the more powerful ingredients. These other components, though they may be less potent, may help to act as buffers, synergists, or counterbalances working in harmony with the more powerful ingredients. Therefore, when you use herbs in their complete form, your body's healing process utilizes a balance of ingredients provided by nature.

In the United States, herbal remedies were used widely until the early 1900s, when what was to become the modern pharmaceutical industry began isolating individual active compounds and producing drugs based on them. American medicine became almost exclusively committed to a medical system some practitioners call *allopathy*, which seeks to treat illness by producing a condition in the body that does not allow the disease to live or thrive. Over the years, most Americans have become conditioned to rely on synthetic, commercial drugs for relief.

Today, however, scientists are taking a second look at herbal remedies. Particularly in the past fifteen years, a growing body of research (much of it done in Europe) has pointed to the therapeutic potential of numerous herbs. But a lot of work remains to be done; only about 15 percent of the estimated plant species on earth have been investigated for possible medicinal uses.

Today's renewed interest in herbs reflects increasing concern about the side effects of powerful synthetic drugs, as well as the desire of many people to take charge of their own health, rather than merely submitting themselves to a sometimes impersonal health care system. We are also rediscovering the healthful benefits of tasty herbs for cooking and aromatic herbs for enhancing and helping to balance mental, spiritual, and physical health.

Nature's pharmacy is an abundant one. Many herbs are rich in compounds that have a beneficial effect on certain tissues and organs, and, therefore, can be used as medicines to treat, cure, or prevent disease. Herbal remedies can help nourish your immune system, stimulate the regeneration of damaged liver tissue, build the strength of the adrenal glands, counter the adverse side effects of chemotherapy, balance the endocrine system, stimulate milk production, and improve night vision, among other things.

Generally, medicinal herbs fall into two basic categories: tonic and stimulating.

Tonics help cells, tissues, and organs to maintain tone, or balance, throughout the body. Some tonics activate and invigorate bodily processes or parts. Other tonics supply important nutrients that cells, tissues, and organs need to function properly. Tonics ordinarily are taken regularly for three to nine months at a time to gently strengthen and improve overall health and/or certain organ functions.

Stimulating herbs have much stronger actions and are used to treat particular ailments. They should be taken in smaller doses than tonic herbs, and for shorter periods of time.

PHYTOMEDICINALS: THE HEALING POWER OF HERBS

Ancient cultures had no idea why herbs worked—they simply knew that certain plants produced certain desired results. Only in the last 100 years or so have chemists and pharmacists been isolating and purifying the beneficial chemical compounds in plants to produce reliable pharmaceutical drugs. About 25 percent of the prescription medicines sold today are (or were originally) derived from plants. For example, morphine and codeine come from the opium poppy; aspirin originated from willow bark; digitalis, a heart muscle strengthener, is derived from the foxglove plant; and paclitaxel (Taxol), used in cancer chemotherapy, comes from the Pacific yew tree.

Phytomedicine, a recently coined term, refers to an herbal medicine that is a whole-plant preparation, rather than a single isolated chemical compound. (The prefix *phyto* comes from the Greek word *phyton,* meaning "plant.") The herbal preparation derived from a whole plant or plant part is considered the active entity, even though it may actually contain hundreds of individual active components. Phytomedicines are standardized, however—that is, they contain set percentages of specified active components—and their therapeutic values are backed by pharmacological and clinical studies and experience.

Phytomedicines are widely recognized in Europe, where they are categorized as plant-derived drugs. In Germany, for example, phytomedicines are considered "ethical drugs," and physicians prescribe them and pharmacists dispense them. In the United States, phytomedicines are sold as over-the-counter dietary supplements in health food stores and in some pharmacies. A few mainstream doctors, however, have begun prescribing herbal remedies along with standard drugs. Some health insurance companies cover the cost of herbal medicines when they are prescribed by health care professionals. And the Office of Alternative Medicine, part of the National Institutes of Health, is funding research on herbal remedies. According to an article published in *USA Today,* nearly 50 million Americans regularly use herbal supplements.

OTHER HERBAL HEALING SYSTEMS

The World Health Organization estimates that 80 percent of the earth's population today depends on plants to treat common ailments. Herbalism is an essential part of Ayurvedic (Indian), traditional Asian, Native American, and naturopathic medicines. Many homeopathic remedies are derived from plants as well.

Oriental herbs are a recent addition to the American herb scene, with the influx of several popular Chinese herbs. The Chinese are today's foremost herbalists, drawing on thousands of years of experience in compounding and processing roots and herbs. In the Asian tradition, herbs are used to bring the whole body into balance and harmony. They are taken daily as a preventive measure, rather than as a treatment once illness has occurred. In the Orient, medicinal herbs often find their way into foods as seasoning and ingredients. Indeed, according to the late Chinese writer and scholar Lin Yutang, the Chinese view medicine and food as the same thing, believing that what is good for the body is medicine and at the same time is also food. Some of the Chinese herbs most readily found in U.S. herb and natural food stores include astragalus, Chinese ginseng, ginkgo biloba, gotu kola, licorice root, dong quai, ginger, and schizandra.

209

Every Native American nation has its own herbal medicine tradition based on the plants growing in the geographic area where it lives. Common among all Native American cultures is the spirituality attached to the gathering and use of herbs, and many peoples use the same herbs both medicinally and ceremonially. For the Navajos, for example, herbalism is a complex and specialized religion, in which the Navajo healer serves as both doctor and priest. Before plants are collected, prayers and offerings are made to the earth and the plant spirit. Herbs used in healing ceremonies are not thrown away, but are reverently placed back into the earth. Much like the Asian approach, Native American herbalism aims to achieve balance within the total person. Medicinal and ceremonial herbs commonly used by Native American cultures include American ginseng, yarrow, black cohosh, boneset, echinacea, goldenseal, nettles, juniper, wild buckwheat, and dogwood.

As they have for centuries, indigenous rainforest tribes around the world rely on the forests for virtually all their medicines. They too have incorporated herbs into their religions and everyday lives. Researchers estimate that the world's rainforests contain literally thousands of potentially useful medicinal plants. Rainforests exist on every continent, though most research attention is currently directed at the rainforests of South America, particularly in the Amazon, and of the South Pacific Islands. Out of this rich storehouse of natural remedies, only a handful are now commonly found in health food stores, among them pau d'arco, boldo, cat's claw, kava, yerba maté, suma, yohimbe, guarana, and passionflower. More and more rainforest remedies are becoming available, however.

USING MEDICINAL HERBS

Commercial herbal preparations are available in several different forms, including bulk herbs, medicinal herb blends, teas, oils, tinctures, fluid extracts, and tablets or capsules. Following are some of the ways in which herbal remedies can be used.

Essential Oils

Essential oils are highly concentrated extracts—typically obtained either by steam distillation or cold pressing—from the flowers, leaves, roots, berries, stems, seeds, gums, needles, bark, or resins of numerous plants. They contain natural hormones, vitamins, antibiotics, and antiseptics. Known also as *volatile oils* because they evaporate easily in air, essential oils are soluble in vegetable oil, partially soluble in alcohol, and not soluble in water. Because they are so concentrated, they are likely to irritate mucous membranes and the stomach lining if taken internally. It is therefore best to use essential oils externally only, such as in poultices, inhalants, bath water, or on the skin (a few drops). The therapeutic properties of essential oils can help to remedy ailments ranging from insomnia to respiratory disorders to impotence to arthritis.

Extracts

An extract is a concentrate that results when crude herb is mixed with a suitable solvent, such as alcohol and/or water. Of the different herbal forms, extracts are generally the most effective because their active ingredients are more highly concentrated, and they can be standardized to a guaranteed potency. Extracts also have longer shelf lives than other herbal preparations. Fresh herbal extracts retain almost all of the original plant's benefits.

Alcohol-free extracts are available. When administered sublingually (drops are placed under the tongue), herbal extracts can be absorbed by the body quickly. This is an especially effective way for older adults and people with absorption problems to use herbs.

Plasters, Compresses, and Poultices

These are ways of applying herbal remedies directly to the skin. Plasters and compresses are cotton bandages soaked in infusions or decoctions and wrapped around the affected area or held on with pressure. Compresses are also warm. Poultices are made by moistening herbs, placing them on the skin, and holding them there with a bandage. Moistened and warmed herbal tea bags also help soothe and heal. Try using chamomile tea bags to relieve the itching and inflammation of insect bites and eczema.

Powders

Powders are dried herbs ground to a fine consistency. You can sprinkle them over food, stir them into a liquid such as juice or water for tonics, or add them to soup stocks. You also can take them in capsule or tablet form.

Salves, Ointments, and Creams

These preparations combine a medicinal herb with an oily base for external use. Creams are light and slightly oily, to blend with the skin's secretions and allow the active ingredients to penetrate the skin. The heavier and oilier salves and ointments apply protective remedies to the skin surface.

Syrups

Syrups are used to improve the taste of bitter herbal formulas and to administer soothing cough or throat medicines. Herbs often taken in syrup form include wild cherry, marshmallow root, and licorice.

Teas, Infusions, and Decoctions

People have been consuming herbal teas for as long as they have known how to heat water—since well before recorded history. Unlike green, black, and oolong teas, herbal teas can be made from virtually any plant, and from any part of the plant, including the roots, flowers, seeds, berries, or bark, although there are some herbs, such as echinacea, gingko leaf, saw palmetto, and milk thistle, that are not effective at healing when taken in tea form because their active components are not water soluble, and the concentration needed for medicinal potency is so high it can be obtained only from an extract, pill, or capsule.

Different herbal teas, which sometimes contain thousands of beneficial active compounds, have their own distinctive healing uses. According to Varro Tyler, Ph.D., distinguished professor emeritus of pharmacognosy (the study of natural drug properties) at Purdue University, herbal teas are very good for relieving mild to moderate ailments such as upset stomach, sore throat, coughs, stuffy nose, and insomnia.

Many herbal teas are available in tea bag form. They can also be prepared from the raw herb. To make an herbal tea, gently crumble leaves and flowers and break roots and barks into pieces (cutting the herbs causes the essential oils to dissipate) and place them in a ceramic or glass container. Cover the herb parts with boiling water (do not bring the herbs themselves to a boil), and allow them to steep. Most herbs should be steeped for four to six minutes, although some herbal teas, such as chamomile, need to be steeped for fifteen to twenty minutes in a covered container in order to deliver their full therapeutic effect. Other herbs, such as ginseng roots, can be boiled. Astragalus can be lightly simmered for several hours. In fact, in Asia, ginseng root, astragalus, dong quai, and other herbs are added to chicken broth to make a tonic soup that is both food and medicine.

Infusion is simply another term for tea. This is the easiest way to take herbal remedies. To make an infusion, you simply boil water and add leaves, stems, flowers, or powdered herbs—plant material whose active ingredients dissolve readily in hot water—then steep, strain, and drink the mixture as a tea.

A decoction is a tea made from thicker plant parts, such as bark, roots, seeds, or berries. These also contain lignin, a substance that is difficult to dissolve in water. Thus, decoctions require a more vigorous extraction method than infusions.

Tinctures

Plant components that are either insoluble or only partially soluble in water can be extracted with solvents such as alcohol or glycerol. The herb is soaked in the solvent for a period of time, then pressed to render the tincture. Tinctures can preserve extracted ingredients for twelve months or more.

Vinegars

Herbal vinegars can serve as both medicines and salad dressings. To make an herbal vinegar, add the herb or herbs of your choice to raw apple cider vinegar, balsamic vinegar, rice vinegar, or malt vinegar. Allow the herbs to steep for four days (agitate the container daily), strain, then press through a straining cloth and bottle in a dark glass container.

Wines

Steeping herbs in wine is a novel and pleasant way to use them medicinally. Wine does not keep as long as the stronger alcohols, so refrigeration is a good idea.

However they are used, most herbs act gently and subtly. They do not produce the kind of dramatic, immediate results we expect from prescription drugs. Basically, herbs are balancers that work with the body to help it heal and regulate itself. They work better together than they do singly because the effect of one herb is usually supported and reinforced when combined with others.

While most herbs aren't likely to be harmful, keep in mind that "natural" isn't a synonym for "safe." Like synthetic drugs, herbal preparations may be toxic, cause allergic reactions, or affect your response to other medications. Common sense, care, and forethought are needed when using herbs for either food or medicine. Here are some essential guidelines for herbal self-care:

- Use herbal self-care for minor ailments only, not for serious or life-threatening conditions.
- Use only recommended amounts for recommended periods of time.
- Use the correct herb. Buy your herbal remedies from a reputable company. If you collect or grow herbs on your own, be absolutely positive in your identification.
- Use the correct part of the plant. For instance, don't substitute roots for leaves. When buying fresh herbs, check to be sure which part of the herb is required for a remedy—the whole herb, flowers, fruit, leaves, stems, or roots.
- When using an herbal remedy for the first time, start with a small amount to test for possible allergic reactions.
- Don't take certain herbs if you are pregnant or planning to become pregnant.
- Don't take herbal remedies if you are nursing a baby.
- Don't give medicinal amounts of herbs to children without first consulting with your health care practitioner.

BUYING HERBAL REMEDIES

When choosing herbal remedies, it is important to select quality products from a reliable source. How do you know whether a manufacturer or supplier is reliable? Start by making a phone call to the manufacturer. Ask how long the company has been in business, what their quality control practices are, and how they determine the identity and potency of the herbs they sell. Membership in trade groups such as the American Herbal Products Association, while not a stamp of approval, does indicate the company's recognition of industry standards. We recommend purchasing herbs sold by reputable companies that have been in the herb business for at least ten years.

If you wish to buy organically grown herbs, look for the "certified organic" label on the product. More than half of U.S. states have certification programs for organic farms and products. Federal standards that will be implemented through a nationwide certification system are now being formulated under the USDA's National Organic Program.

Finally, look for herbal products that are standardized to contain a specific percentage of active ingredient extracted from the specific herb part known to be effective.

HERBS AND THEIR USES

Acerola (Malpighia glabra)

PARTS USED Fruit.

PHYTOCHEMICAL AND NUTRIENT CONTENT Phytochemicals: Beta-carotene. Nutrients: Calcium, iron, magnesium, phosphorus, potassium, vitamins A, B_1, B_2, B_3, B_5, B_6, and C.

ACTIONS AND USES Has antioxidant, antifungal, and astringent properties. Helps to support the liver and hydrate the skin. Useful for diarrhea and fever.

COMMENTS A rainforest herb similar to the cherry. One of the richest natural sources of vitamin C; found in numerous multivitamin supplements.

Alfalfa (Medicago sativa)

PARTS USED Flowers, leaves, petals, sprouted seeds.

PHYTOCHEMICAL AND NUTRIENT CONTENT Phytochemicals: Alpha-carotene, beta-carotene, beta-sitosterol, chlorophyll, coumarin, cryptoxanthin, daidzein, fumaric acid, genistein, limonene, lutein, saponin, stigmasterol, zeaxanthin. Nutrients: Calcium, copper, fo-

215

late, iron, magnesium, manganese, phosphorus, potassium, silicon, zinc, vitamins A, B_1, B_2, B_3, B_5, B_6, C, D, E, and K.

ACTIONS AND USES Alkalizes and detoxifies the body. Acts as a diuretic, anti-inflammatory, and antifungal. Lowers cholesterol, balances blood sugar and hormones, and promotes pituitary gland function. Good for anemia, arthritis, ulcers, bleeding-related disorders, and disorders of the bones and joints, digestive system, and skin.

COMMENTS Must be used in fresh, raw form to provide all nutrients. Sprouts are especially effective (be sure to rinse them thoroughly before use to remove mold and bacteria).

Aloe (*Aloe vera*)

PARTS USED Pulp from insides of succulent leaves.

PHYTOCHEMICAL AND NUTRIENT CONTENT Phytochemicals: Acemannan, beta-carotene, beta-sitosterol, campesterol, cinnamic acid, coumarin, lignins, p-coumaric acid, saponins. Nutrients: Amino acids, calcium, folate, iron, magnesium, phosphorus, potassium, zinc, vitamins A, B_1, B_2, B_3, C, and E.

ACTIONS AND USES Acts as an astringent, emollient, antifungal, antibacterial, and antiviral. Applied topically, heals burns and wounds; and stimulates cell regeneration. Ingested, helps to lower cholesterol, reduces inflammation resulting from radiation therapy, increases blood-vessel generation in lower extremities of people with poor circulation, soothes stomach irritation, aids healing, and acts as a laxative. Good for AIDS and for skin and digestive disorders.

COMMENTS Allergic reactions, though rare, may occur in susceptible persons. Before using, apply a small amount behind the ear or on the underarm. If stinging or rash occurs, do not use. *Caution:* Should not be taken internally during pregnancy.

Anise (*Pimpinella anisum*)

PARTS USED Seeds, seed oil.

PHYTOCHEMICAL AND NUTRIENT CONTENT Phytochemicals: Alpha-pinene, apigenin, bergapten, caffeic acid, chlorogenic acid, eugenol, limonene, linalool, myristicin, rutin, scopoletin, squalene, stigmasterol, umbelliferone. Nutrients: Calcium, iron, magnesium, manganese, phosphorus, potassium, zinc, vitamins A, B_1, B_2, B_3, B_5, B_6, C, and E.

ACTIONS AND USES Aids digestion, clears mucus from air passages, combats infection, and promotes milk production in nursing mothers. Good for indigestion and for respiratory infections such as sinusitis. Also helpful for menopausal symptoms.

COMMENTS Used in many popular products as a fragrance and flavoring.

Annatto (*Bixa orellana*)

217

PARTS USED Leaves, roots, seeds.

PHYTOCHEMICAL AND NUTRIENT CONTENT Phytochemicals: Beta-carotene, bixin, cyanidin, ellagic acid, salicylic acid, saponin, tannins. Nutrients: Amino acids, calcium, iron, phosphorus, vitamins B_2, B_3, and C.

ACTIONS AND USES Has diuretic, antioxidant, antibacterial, anti-inflammatory, and expectorant properties. Helps to protect the liver and kidneys. May reduce blood sugar levels. Useful for indigestion, fever, coughs, burns, skin problems, and weight loss.

COMMENTS A rainforest herb used in skin care products as an emollient, and as an orange-yellow food coloring.

Ashwagandha (*Withania somnifera*)

PARTS USED Roots.

PHYTOCHEMICAL AND NUTRIENT CONTENT Phytochemicals: Alkaloids, beta-sitosterol, chlorogenic acid, scopoletin, withaferin. Nutrients: Amino acids, choline.

ACTIONS AND USES Rejuvenates and energizes the nervous system. Helps prevent stress-related disorders and stress-related depletion of vitamin C and cortisol. Increases physical endurance and improves sexual function. Has anti-inflammatory and anti-aging effects. In laboratory studies, has modulated and stimulated immune function.

COMMENTS An Ayurvedic herb also known as Indian ginseng and winter cherry. An important herb in Ayurvedic medicine.

Astragalus (Astragalus membranaceus)

PARTS USED Roots.

PHYTOCHEMICAL AND NUTRIENT CONTENT Phytochemicals: Betaine, beta-sitosterol, formononetin, isoliquiritigenin. Nutrients: Calcium, choline, copper, essential fatty acids, iron, magnesium, manganese, potassium, zinc.

ACTIONS AND USES Acts as a tonic to protect the immune system. Aids adrenal gland function and digestion. Increases metabolism, produces spontaneous sweating, promotes healing, and provides energy to combat fatigue and prolonged stress. Increases stamina. Good for colds, flu, and immune-deficiency-related problems, including AIDS, cancer, and tumors. Effective for chronic lung weakness.

COMMENTS Also called huang qi. *Caution:* Should not be taken if fever is present.

Barberry (Berberis vulgaris)

PARTS USED Bark, berries, roots.

PHYTOCHEMICAL AND NUTRIENT CONTENT Phytochemicals: Berbamine, berberine, beta-carotene, caffeic acid, kaempferol, lutein, quercetin, sinapic acid, zeaxanthin. Nutrients: Calcium, iron, magnesium, manganese, phosphorus, potassium, selenium, silicon, zinc, vitamins B_1, B_2, B_3, and C.

ACTIONS AND USES Decreases heart rate, slows breathing, reduces bronchial constriction. Kills bacteria on the skin and stimulates intestinal movement.

COMMENTS *Caution:* Should not be used during pregnancy.

Bayberry *(Myrica cerifera)*

PARTS USED Root bark.

PHYTOCHEMICAL AND NUTRIENT CONTENT Phytochemicals: Beta-carotene, gallic acid, myristic acid, phenol. Nutrients: Calcium, iron, magnesium, manganese, phosphorus, potassium, selenium, silicon, zinc, vitamins B_1, B_2, B_3, and C.

ACTIONS AND USES Acts as a decongestant and astringent. Aids circulation, reduces fever. Helps stop bleeding. Good for circulatory disorders, fever, hypothyroidism, and ulcers. Also good for the eyes and the immune system.

COMMENTS The wax of the berries is used to make fragrant candles. *Caution:* Should not be used at high dosages or for prolonged periods. May temporarily irritate sensitive stomachs.

Bilberry *(Vaccinium myrtillus)*

PARTS USED Entire plant.

PHYTOCHEMICAL AND NUTRIENT CONTENT Phytochemicals: Anthocyanosides, beta-carotene, caffeic acid, caryophyllene, catechin, chlorogenic acid, ferulic acid, gallic acid, hyperoside, lutein, quercetin, quercitrin, ursolic acid, vanillic acid. Nutrients: Calcium, inositol, magnesium, manganese, phosphorus, potassium, selenium, silicon, sulfur, zinc, vitamins B_1, B_2, B_3, and C.

ACTIONS AND USES Acts as an antioxidant, diuretic, and urinary tract antiseptic. Keeps blood vessels flexible, allowing increased blood flow. Helps control insulin levels and strengthen connective tissue. Supports and strengthens collagen structures, inhibits the growth of bacteria, and has anti-aging and anticarcinogenic effects. Useful for hypoglycemia, inflammation, stress, anxiety, night blindness, and cataracts. May help halt or prevent macular degeneration.

COMMENTS Also known as European blueberry. Related to the American blueberry. *Caution:* Interferes with iron absorption when taken internally. Should not be used by people with diabetes except under the supervision of a knowledgable health professional.

Birch (*Betula alba*)

PARTS USED Bark, leaves, sap.

PHYTOCHEMICAL AND NUTRIENT CONTENT Phytochemicals: Betulin, betulinic acid, hyperoside, luteolin and quercetin glycosides, methyl salicylate.

ACTIONS AND USES Acts as a diuretic, anti-inflammatory, and pain reliever. Good for joint pain and urinary tract infections. Applied topically, good for boils and sores.

COMMENTS Betulinic acid in birch bark has been found to kill cancer cells.

Black cohosh (*Cimicifuga racemosa*)

PARTS USED Rhizomes, roots.

PHYTOCHEMICAL AND NUTRIENT CONTENT Phytochemicals: Beta-carotene, cimicifugin, formononetin, gallic acid, phytosterols, salicylic acid, tannic acid, tannin. Nutrients: Calcium, chromium, iron, magnesium, manganese, phosphorus, potassium, selenium, silicon, zinc, vitamins B_1, B_2, B_3, and C.

ACTIONS AND USES Lowers blood pressure and cholesterol levels. Reduces mucus production. Helps cardiovascular and circulatory disorders. Induces labor and aids in childbirth (many herbalists recommend taking small amounts 2 weeks before expected delivery). Relieves menopausal symptoms, menstrual cramps with back pain, morning sickness, and pain. Helpful for poisonous snake bites. Good for arthritis.

COMMENTS Also known as black snakeroot. *Caution:* Should not be used during pregnancy (until just before birth) or in the presence of chronic disease.

Black walnut (*Juglans nigra*)

PARTS USED Husks, inner bark, leaves, nuts.

PHYTOCHEMICAL AND NUTRIENT CONTENT Phytochemicals: Beta-carotene, ellagic acid, juglone, myricetin, tannin. Nutrients: Calcium, iron, magnesium, manganese, phosphorus, potassium, selenium, silicon, zinc, vitamins B_1, B_2, B_3, and C.

ACTIONS AND USES Aids digestion and acts as a laxative. Helps heal mouth and throat sores. Cleanses the body of some types of parasites. Good for bruising, fungal infection, herpes, poison ivy, and warts. May help lower blood pressure and cholesterol levels.

COMMENTS When boiled, the hulls produce a dye that is used to color wool.

Blessed thistle (*Cnicus benedictus*)

PARTS USED Flowers, leaves, stems.

PHYTOCHEMICAL AND NUTRIENT CONTENT Phytochemicals: Beta-carotene, beta-sitosterol, cnicin, ferulic acid, kaempferol, luteolin, oleanolic acid, stigmasterol. Nutrients: Calcium, essential fatty acids, iron, magnesium, manganese, phosphorus, potassium, selenium, silicon, zinc, vitamins B_1, B_2, B_3, and C.

ACTIONS AND USES Stimulates the appetite and stomach secretions. Heals the liver. Lessens inflammation, improves circulation, cleanses the blood, and strengthens the heart. May act as brain food. Good for female disorders and increases milk flow in nursing mothers.

COMMENTS Also called St. Benedict thistle, holy thistle. *Caution:* Should be handled with care to avoid toxic skin effects.

Blue cohosh (*Caulophyllum thalictroides*)

PARTS USED Roots.

PHYTOCHEMICAL AND NUTRIENT CONTENT Phytochemicals: Anagyrine, beta-carotene, caulophylline, caulophyllosaponin, caulosaponin, hederagenin, phytosterols, saponin. Nutrients: Calcium,

221

iron, magnesium, manganese, phosphorus, potassium, selenium, zinc, vitamins B_1, B_2, B_3, and C.

ACTIONS AND USES Eases muscle spasms and stimulates uterine contractions for childbirth. Useful for memory problems, menstrual disorders, and nervous disorders.

COMMENTS *Caution:* Should not be used during the first two trimesters of pregnancy.

Boldo (Peumus boldus)

PARTS USED Leaves.

PHYTOCHEMICAL AND NUTRIENT CONTENT Phytochemicals: Alpha-pinene, ascaridole, benzaldehyde, beta-pinene, boldin, boldine, camphor, coumarin, eugenol, farnesol, kaempferol, limonene, linalool, 1,8-cineole. Nutrients: Choline.

ACTIONS AND USES Acts as a diuretic, laxative, antibiotic, liver tonic, and anti-inflammatory. Aids in the excretion of uric acid and stimulates digestion.

COMMENTS Used by indigenous peoples of Chile and Peru for liver ailments and gallstones.

Boneset (Eupatorium perfoliatum)

PARTS USED Flower petals, leaves.

PHYTOCHEMICAL AND NUTRIENT CONTENT Phytochemicals: Astragalin, gallic acid, eufoliatin, eufoliatorin, eupatorin, euperfolin, euperfolitin, gallic acid, hyperoside, kaempferol, quercetin, rutin, tannic acid.

ACTIONS AND USES Acts as a decongestant, laxative, anti-inflammatory, and diuretic. Loosens phlegm, reduces fever, increases perspiration, calms the body. Useful for colds, flu, bronchitis, and fever-induced aches and pains.

COMMENTS Also called white snakeroot. *Caution:* Long-term use should be avoided, as it can result in toxicity.

Borage *(Borago officinalis)*

PARTS USED Leaves, seeds.

PHYTOCHEMICAL AND NUTRIENT CONTENT Phytochemicals: Beta-carotene, rosmarinic acid, silicic acid, tannin. Nutrients: Calcium, choline, essential fatty acids, iron, magnesium, phosphorus, potassium, zinc, vitamins B_1, B_2, B_3, and C.

ACTIONS AND USES Acts as an adrenal tonic and gland balancer. Contains valuable minerals and essential fatty acids needed for proper cardiovascular function and healthy skin and nails.

COMMENTS The flowers of the borage plant are edible.

Boswellia *(Boswellia serrata)*

PARTS USED Gum resin.

PHYTOCHEMICAL AND NUTRIENT CONTENT Phytochemicals: Borneol, boswellic acids, carvone, caryophyllene, farnesol, geraniol, limonene.

ACTIONS AND USES Acts as an anti-inflammatory, anti-arthritic, antifungal, and antibacterial. Used topically for pain relief. Lowers cholesterol, protects the liver. Useful for arthritis, gout, low back pain, myositis, and fibromyalgia. Helps repair blood vessels damaged by inflammation. Traditionally used as a remedy for obesity, diarrhea, dysentery, pulmonary diseases, ringworm, and boils.

COMMENTS An Ayurvedic herb also known as Indian frankincense. An important herb in Ayurvedic medicine.

Buchu *(Barosma betulina)*

PARTS USED Leaves.

PHYTOCHEMICAL AND NUTRIENT CONTENT Phytochemicals: Alpha-pinene, alpha-terpinene, barosma-camphor, diosphenol, hesperidin, limonene, menthone, pulegone, quercetin, quercetrin, rutin. Nutrients: Calcium, iron, magnesium, manganese, phosphorus, potassium, selenium, silicon, zinc, vitamins B_1, B_2, and B_3.

ACTIONS AND USES Lessens inflammation of the colon, gums, mucous membranes, prostate, sinuses, and vagina. Acts as a diuretic. Helps control bladder and kidney problems, diabetes, digestive disorders, fluid retention, and prostate disorders. A specific for bladder infections.

COMMENTS Do not boil buchu leaves.

Burdock (Arctium lappa)

PARTS USED Plant, roots, seeds.

PHYTOCHEMICAL AND NUTRIENT CONTENT Phytochemicals: Acetic acid, arctigenin, arctiin, beta-carotene, butyric acid, caffeic acid, chlorogenic acid, costic acid, inulin, isovaleric acid, lauric acid, lignin, myristic acid, propionic acid, sitosterol, stigmasterol. Nutrients: Amino acids, calcium, copper, chromium, iron, magnesium, manganese, phosphorus, potassium, selenium, silicon, zinc, vitamins B_1, B_2, B_3, and C.

ACTIONS AND USES Acts as an antioxidant. May help to protects against cancer by helping control cell mutation. Aids elimination of excess fluid, uric acid, and toxins. Has antibacterial and antifungal properties. Purifies the blood, restores liver and gallbladder function, and stimulates the digestive and immune systems. Helps skin disorders such as boils and carbuncles, and relieves gout and menopausal symptoms. Burdock root used as a hair rinse promotes scalp and hair health.

COMMENTS *Caution:* Interferes with iron absorption when taken internally.

Butcher's broom (Ruscus aculeatus)

PARTS USED Plant, roots, seeds.

PHYTOCHEMICAL AND NUTRIENT CONTENT Phytochemicals: Beta-carotene, chrysophanic acid, glycolic acid, neoruscogenin, rutin, saponin. Nutrients: Calcium, chromium, iron, magnesium, manganese, phosphorus, potassium, selenium, silicon, zinc, vitamins B_1, B_2, B_3, and C.

ACTIONS AND USES Reduces inflammation. Useful for carpal tunnel syndrome, circulatory disorders, edema, Ménière's disease, obesity, Raynaud's phenomenon, thrombophlebitis, varicose veins, and vertigo. Also good for the bladder and kidneys.

COMMENTS More effective if taken with vitamin C.

Calendula (*Calendula officinalis*)

PARTS USED Flower petals.

PHYTOCHEMICAL AND NUTRIENT CONTENT Phytochemicals: Alpha-amyrin, beta-amyrin, beta-sitosterol, caffeic acid, campesterol, caryophyllene, chlorogenic acid, faradiol, galactose, gentisic acid, kaempferol, lutein, lycopene, malic acid, myristic acid, oleanolic acid, p-coumaric acid, phytofluene, quercetin, rutin, salicylic acid, saponin, stigmasterol, syringic acid, taraxasterol vanillic acid, zeta-carotene. Nutrients: Calcium, coenzyme Q_{10}, vitamins C and E.

ACTIONS AND USES Reduces inflammation and is soothing to the skin. Helps regulate the menstrual cycle and lower fever. Useful for skin disorders, such as rashes and sunburn, as well as for neuritis and toothache. Good for diaper rash and other skin problems in small children.

225

COMMENTS Also called pot marigold. Usually nonirritating when used externally.

Cascara sagrada (*Frangula purshiana*)

PARTS USED Bark.

PHYTOCHEMICAL AND NUTRIENT CONTENT Phytochemicals: Aloe-emodin, anthraquinones, barbaloin, beta-carotene, casanthranol, chrysophanic acid, chrysophanol, frangulin, malic acid, myristic acid. Nutrients: Calcium, iron, linoleic acid, magnesium, manganese, phosphorus, potassium, selenium, silicon, zinc, vitamins B_1, B_2, B_3, and C.

ACTIONS AND USES Acts as a colon cleanser and laxative. Effective for colon disorders, constipation, and parasitic infestation.

COMMENTS Tastes very bitter taken as a tea.

Catnip (Nepeta cataria)

PARTS USED Leaves.

PHYTOCHEMICAL AND NUTRIENT CONTENT Phytochemicals: Alpha-humulene, beta-elemene, camphor, carvacrol, caryophyllene, citral, citronellal, geraniol, myrcene, nepetalactone, piperitone, pulegone, rosmarinic acid, thymol. Nutrients: Calcium, chromium, iron, magnesium, manganese, phosphorus, potassium, selenium, silicon, zinc.

ACTIONS AND USES Lowers fever (catnip tea enemas reduce fever quickly). Dispels gas and aids digestion and sleep; relieves stress; stimulates the appetite. Good for anxiety, colds and flu, inflammation, pain, and stress.

COMMENTS Can be given to children.

Cat's claw (Uncaria tomentosa)

PARTS USED Inner bark, roots.

PHYTOCHEMICAL AND NUTRIENT CONTENT Phytochemicals: Alloisopteropodine, allopteropodine, isomitraphylline, isopteropodine, mitraphylline, oleanolic acid, pteropodine, rhynchophylline, ursolic acid.

ACTIONS AND USES Acts as an antioxidant and anti-inflammatory. Stimulates the immune system. Cleanses the intestinal tract and enhances the action of white blood cells. Good for intestinal problems and viral infections. May help people with AIDS, arthritis, cancer, tumors, or ulcers.

COMMENTS Also called uña de gato. According to USDA research, cat's claw seeds contain an enzyme instrumental in converting saturated fats to unsaturated fats. *Caution:* Should not be used during pregnancy.

Cayenne (Capsicum frutescens or C. annum)

PARTS USED Berries.

PHYTOCHEMICAL AND NUTRIENT CONTENT Phytochemicals: Alpha-carotene, beta-carotene, beta-ionone, caffeic acid, campesterol, capsaicin, carvone, caryophyllene, chlorogenic acid, citric acid, cryptoxanthin, hesperidin, kaempferol, limonene, lutein, myristic acid, 1,8-cineole, p-coumaric acid, quercetin, scopoletin, stigmasterol, zeaxanthin. Nutrients: Amino acids, calcium, essential fatty acids, folate, iron, magnesium, phosphorus, potassium, zinc, vitamins B_1, B_2, B_3, B_5, B_6, C, and E.

ACTIONS AND USES Aids digestion, improves circulation, and stops bleeding from ulcers. Acts as a catalyst for other herbs. Good for the heart, kidneys, lungs, pancreas, spleen, and stomach. Useful for arthritis and rheumatism. Helps to ward off colds, sinus infections, and sore throats. Good for pain when applied topically. Used with lobelia for nerves.

COMMENTS Also called capsicum, hot pepper, red pepper. *Caution:* Avoid contact with the eyes.

Cedar (Cedrus libani)

PARTS USED Leaves, tops.

PHYTOCHEMICAL AND NUTRIENT CONTENT Phytochemicals: Borneol, quinic acid.

ACTIONS AND USES Acts as an antiviral, antifungal, expectorant, lymphatic cleanser, and urinary antiseptic. Stimulates the immune system. Increases venous blood flow. Can be used externally for warts.

Celery (Apium graveolens)

PARTS USED Plant, roots, seeds.

PHYTOCHEMICAL AND NUTRIENT CONTENT Phytochemicals: Alphapinene, apigenin, bergapten, beta-carotene, caffeic acid, carvone, chlorogenic acid, coumarin, eugenol, ferulic acid, isoquercitrin, limonene, linalool, luteolin, mannitol, myristic acid, myristicin, p-coumaric acid, rutin, scopoletin, shikimic acid, thymol. Nutrients: Amino acids, boron, calcium, choline, essential fatty acids, folate, inositol, iron, magnesium, manganese, phosphorus, potassium, selenium, sulfur, zinc, vitamins A, B_1, B_2, B_3, B_5, B_6, C, E, and K.

ACTIONS AND USES Reduces blood pressure, relieves muscle spasms, and improves appetite. Good for arthritis, gout, and kidney problems. Acts as an diuretic, antioxidant, and sedative.

COMMENTS *Caution:* The seeds should not be used during pregnancy, nor should large amounts of the herb.

Chamomile *(Matricaria recutita or M. chamomilla)*

PARTS USED Flowers, plant.

PHYTOCHEMICAL AND NUTRIENT CONTENT Phytochemicals: Alpha-bisabolol, apigenin, azulene, borneol, caffeic acid, chlorogenic acid, farnesol, gentisic acid, geraniol, hyperoside, kaempferol, luteolin, p-coumaric acid, perillyl alcohol, quercetin, rutin, salicylic acid, sinapic acid, tannin, umbelliferone. Nutrients: Choline, vitamins B_1, B_3, and C.

ACTIONS AND USES Reduces inflammation, stimulates the appetite, and aids digestion and sleep. Acts as a diuretic and nerve tonic. Helpful for colitis, diverticulosis, fever, headaches, and pain. Good for menstrual cramps. A traditional remedy for stress and anxiety, indigestion, and insomnia. Useful as a mouthwash for minor mouth and gum infections.

COMMENTS Also called German chamomile, wild chamomile. Roman chamomile *(Chamaemelum nobile)* is also available, but is less common. *Caution:* Should not be used daily for long periods of time, as this may lead to ragweed allergy. Should be used with caution by those who are allergic to ragweed. Should not be used with sedatives or alcohol.

Chanca piedra *(Phyllanthus niruri)*

PARTS USED Entire plant.

PHYTOCHEMICAL AND NUTRIENT CONTENT Phytochemicals: Limonene, lupeol, methyl salicylate, quercetin, quercitrin, rutin, saponins.

ACTIONS AND USES Fights inflammation and bacterial and viral infection. Acts as a diuretic. Useful for kidney stones, gallstones, colds, flu, digestion, asthma, bronchitis, diarrhea, pain relief, fever, sexually transmitted diseases, and muscle spasms.

COMMENTS A rainforest herb whose name means "stone crusher." Also known as seed-on-the-leaf.

Chaparral (*Larrea tridentata*)

PARTS USED Leaves.

PHYTOCHEMICAL AND NUTRIENT CONTENT Phytochemicals: Alpha-pinene, beta-carotene, borneol, camphene, camphor, gossypetin, limonene, nordihydroguaiaretic acid. Nutrients: Amino acids, calcium, magnesium, selenium, sulfur, zinc, vitamins B_1, B_2, B_3, and C.

ACTIONS AND USES Fights free radicals and chelates heavy metals. Has anti-HIV activity. Protects against harmful effects of radiation, sun exposure, and the formation of tumors and cancer cells. Relieves pain. Good for skin disorders.

COMMENTS *Caution:* Recommended for external use only. Taken internally, especially in large doses and/or for prolonged periods, can cause liver damage.

Chaste tree (*Vitex agnus-castus*)

PARTS USED Fruit, leaf.

PHYTOCHEMICAL AND NUTRIENT CONTENT Phytochemicals: Alpha-pinene, alpha-terpineol, chrysosplenol, flavonoids, limonene, linalool, myrcene, 1,8-cineole, pinene, progesterone, testosterone.

ACTIONS AND USES Has a calming and soothing effect. Relieves muscle cramps. Regulates and normalizes hormone levels and menstrual cycles. Increases and improves breast milk. Good for symptoms of PMS and menopause.

COMMENTS Also called chasteberry, vitex. *Caution:* Should not be used during pregnancy. Should not be given to children.

Chickweed *(Stellaria media)*

PARTS USED Leaves, stems.

PHYTOCHEMICAL AND NUTRIENT CONTENT Phytochemicals: Beta-carotene, genistein, rutin. Nutrients: Calcium, essential fatty acids, iron, magnesium, manganese, phosphorus, potassium, selenium, silicon, sulfur, zinc, vitamins B_1, B_2, B_3, C, and E.

ACTIONS AND USES Relieves nasal congestion. May lower blood lipids. Useful for bronchitis, circulatory problems, colds, coughs, skin diseases, and warts (applied topically). A good source of vitamin C and other nutrients.

COMMENTS Also called starweed.

Chuchuhuasi *(Maytenus krukovit)*

PARTS USED Bark.

PHYTOCHEMICAL AND NUTRIENT CONTENT Anthocyanidins, catechin, maytensine, nocotinyl, sesquiterpenes, triterpenes, tannins.

ACTIONS AND USES Fights inflammation and stimulates the immune system. Supports the adrenal system and balances and regulates menstrual cycles. Good for arthritis, rheumatism, back pain, muscle spasms, fever, skin tumors, bronchitis, diarrhea.

COMMENTS A rainforest herb used traditionally to stimulate sexual desire.

Cinnamon *(Cinnamomum verum)*

PARTS USED Bark, plant.

PHYTOCHEMICAL AND NUTRIENT CONTENT Phytochemicals: Alpha-pinene, benzaldehyde, beta-carotene, beta-pinene, borneol, camphor, caryophyllene, cinnamaldehyde, coumarin, cuminaldehyde, eugenol, farnesol, geraniol, limonene, linalool, mannitol, mucilage, 1,8-cineole, phellandrene, tannin, terpinolene, vanillin. Nutrients: Calcium, chromium, copper, iodine, iron, manganese, phosphorus, potassium, zinc, vitamins A, B_1, B_2, B_3, and C.

ACTIONS AND USES Relieves diarrhea and nausea; counteracts congestion; aids peripheral circulation. Warms the body and enhances digestion, especially the metabolism of fats. Also fights fungal infection. Useful for diabetes, weight loss, yeast infection, and uterine hemorrhaging.

COMMENTS *Caution:* Should not be used in large amounts during pregnancy.

Clove *(Syzygium aromaticum)*

PARTS USED Flower buds, essential oil.

PHYTOCHEMICAL AND NUTRIENT CONTENT Phytochemicals: Beta-carotene, beta-pinene, beta-sitosterol, campesterol, carvone, caryophyllene, chavicol, cinnamaldehyde, ellagic acid, eugenol, gallic acid, kaempferol, linalool, methyleugenol, methylsalicylate, mucilage, oleanolic acid, stigmasterol, tannin, vanillin. Nutrients: Calcium, iron, magnesium, manganese, phosphorus, potassium, zinc, vitamins A, B_1, B_2, and C.

ACTIONS AND USES Has antiseptic and antiparasitic properties, and acts as a digestive aid. Essential oil is applied topically for relief of toothache and mouth pain.

COMMENTS *Caution:* Clove oil is very strong and can cause irritation if used in its pure form. Diluting the oil in olive oil or distilled water is recommended. Essential oil should not be taken internally except under the careful supervision of a health care professional.

Comfrey *(Symphytum officinale)*

PARTS USED Leaves, roots.

PHYTOCHEMICAL AND NUTRIENT CONTENT Phytochemicals: Allantoin, beta-carotene, caffeic acid, chlorogenic acid, rosmarinic acid, sitosterol, stigmasterol. Nutrients: Calcium, iron, magnesium, manganese, phosphorus, potassium, selenium, zinc, vitamins B_1, B_2, B_3, and C.

ACTIONS AND USES Speeds healing of wounds and many skin conditions. Beneficial for bedsores, bites and stings, bruises, inflamed bunions, burns, dermatitis, dry skin, bleeding hemorrhoids, leg ulcers, nosebleeds, psoriasis, scabies, skin rashes, and sunburn.

COMMENTS Also called knitbone. *Caution:* May cause liver damage if taken internally. Not recommended for internal use except under the careful supervision of a health care professional. External use is generally considered safe. Should not be used during pregnancy.

Corn silk (*Zea mays*)

PARTS USED Styles, stigmas ("tassels").

PHYTOCHEMICAL AND NUTRIENT CONTENT Phytochemicals: Benzaldehyde, beta-carotene, betaine, beta-sitosterol, caffeic acid, campesterol, carvacrol, caryophyllene, dioxycinnamic acid, geraniol, glycolic acid, limonene, 1,8-cineole, saponin, thymol, vitexin. Nutrients: Calcium, chromium, iron, magnesium, manganese, phosphorus, potassium, vitamins B_1, B_3, and C.

ACTIONS AND USES Acts as a diuretic. Aids the bladder, kidney, and small intestine. Lessens the incidence of bed-wetting when taken several hours before bedtime. Good for carpal tunnel syndrome, edema, obesity, premenstrual syndrome, and prostate disorders. Used in combination with other "kidney herbs," opens the urinary tract and removes mucus from the urine.

Cramp bark (*Viburnum opulus*)

PARTS USED Bark, root.

PHYTOCHEMICAL AND NUTRIENT CONTENT Phytochemicals: Esculetin, scopoletin, valerianic acid. Nutrients: Calcium, iron, magnesium, manganese, phosphorus, potassium, selenium, zinc.

ACTIONS AND USES Relieves muscle spasms and pain. Good for menstrual cramps. Useful for lower back and leg spasms.

COMMENTS Also called guelder rose. Closely related to black haw, which has the same medicinal properties. *Caution:* Should be avoided during pregnancy.

Cranberry *(Vaccinium macrocarpon)*

PARTS USED Fruit.

PHYTOCHEMICAL AND NUTRIENT CONTENT Phytochemicals: Alpha-terpineol, anthocyanosides, benzaldehyde, benzoic acid, beta-carotene, chlorogenic acid, ellagic acid, eugenol, ferulic acid, lutein, malic acid, quercetin. Nutrients: Calcium, folate, iron, magnesium, manganese, phosphorus, potassium, selenium, sulfur, zinc, vitamins A, B_1, B_2, B_3, B_5, C, and E.

ACTIONS AND USES Acidifies the urine and prevents bacteria from adhering to bladder cells. Good for the kidneys, bladder, and skin. Has anticancer properties. Helpful for infections of the urinary tract.

COMMENTS A good source of vitamin C. Cranberry juice cocktail products that contain sugar should be *avoided.*

Damiana *(Turnera diffusa)*

PARTS USED Leaves.

PHYTOCHEMICAL AND NUTRIENT CONTENT Phytochemicals: Alpha-pinene, beta-carotene, beta-pinene, beta-sitosterol, 1,8-cineole, tannins, thymol. Nutrients: Calcium, iron, magnesium, manganese, phosphorus, potassium, selenium, zinc, vitamins B_1, B_2, B_3, and C.

ACTIONS AND USES Stimulates muscular contractions of the intestinal tract and delivery of oxygen to the genital area. Used as an energy tonic and aphrodisiac, and to remedy sexual and hormonal problems. A "sexuality tonic" for women.

COMMENTS *Caution:* Interferes with iron absorption when taken internally.

Dandelion *(Taraxacum officinale)*

PARTS USED Flowers, leaves, roots, tops.

PHYTOCHEMICAL AND NUTRIENT CONTENT Phytochemicals: Beta-carotene, beta-sitosterol, caffeic acid, cryptoxanthin, lutein, mannitol, p-coumaric acid, saponin, stigmasterol. Nutrients: Calcium, iron, magnesium, manganese, phosphorus, potassium, selenium, zinc, vitamins B_1, B_2, B_3, and C.

ACTIONS AND USES Acts as a diuretic. Cleanses the blood and liver, and increases bile production. Reduces serum cholesterol and uric acid levels. Improves functioning of the kidneys, pancreas, spleen, and stomach. Relieves menopausal symptoms. Useful for abscesses, anemia, boils, breast tumors, cirrhosis of the liver, constipation, fluid retention, hepatitis, jaundice, and rheumatism. Believed to help prevent age spots and breast cancer.

COMMENTS Leaves can be boiled and eaten like spinach (young leaves can be used in salads). *Caution:* Should not be combined with prescription diuretics. Not recommended for people with gallstones or biliary tract obstruction.

Devil's claw *(Harpagophytum procumbens)*

PARTS USED Rhizome.

PHYTOCHEMICAL AND NUTRIENT CONTENT Phytochemicals: Chlorogenic acid, cinnamic acid, harpagide, harpagoside, kaempferol, luteolin, oleanolic acid. Nutrients: Calcium, iron, magnesium, manganese, phosphorus, potassium, selenium, zinc.

ACTIONS AND USES Relieves pain and reduces inflammation. Acts as a diuretic, sedative, and digestive stimulant. Good for back pain; arthritis; rheumatism; diabetes; allergies; liver; gallbladder and kidney disorders; arteriosclerosis; lumbago; gout; and menopausal symptoms.

COMMENTS Also called grapple plant, wood spider. *Caution:* Should not be used during pregnancy.

Dong quai *(Angelica sinensis)*

PARTS USED Roots.

PHYTOCHEMICAL AND NUTRIENT CONTENT Phytochemicals: Alpha-pinene, bergapten, beta-carotene, beta-sitosterol, carvacrol, falcarinol, ferulic acid, ligustilide, myristic acid, p-cymene, scopoletin, umbelliferone, vanillic acid. Nutrients: Calcium, folate, iron, magnesium, manganese, phosphorus, potassium, selenium, zinc, vitamins B_1, B_2, B_5, and C.

ACTIONS AND USES Acts as a mild sedative, laxative, diuretic, antispasmodic, and pain-reliever. Improves the blood. Strengthens the reproductive system. Assists the body in using hormones. Used to treat female problems such as hot flashes and other menopausal symptoms, premenstrual syndrome, and vaginal dryness.

COMMENTS Also known as Chinese angelica. *Caution:* Should not be used during pregnancy. Should not be used by people who have diabetes or are light-sensitive.

Echinacea *(Echinacea species)*

PARTS USED Leaves, roots.

PHYTOCHEMICAL AND NUTRIENT CONTENT Phytochemicals: Alphapinene, apigenin, arabinogalactan, beta-carotene, beta-sitosterol, betaine, borneol, caffeic acid, caryophyllene, chlorogenic acid, cichoric acid, cynarin, echinacoside, ferulic acid, kaempferol, luteolin, quercetin, rutin, stigmasterol, vanillin, verbascoside. Nutrients: Calcium, iron, magnesium, manganese, phosphorus, potassium, selenium, zinc, vitamins B_1, B_2, B_3, and C.

235

ACTIONS AND USES Fights inflammation and bacterial and viral infection. Stimulates certain white blood cells. Good for the immune system and the lymphatic system. Useful for allergies, colic, colds, flu, and other infectious illnesses. Also helpful for snakebite.

COMMENTS For internal use, a freeze-dried form or alcohol-free extract is recommended. *Caution:* Should be used with caution by people who are allergic to ragweed or to plants in the sunflower family. Should not be taken for prolonged periods by people with autoimmune disorders, as it stimulates the immune system.

Elder *(Sambucus nigra)*

PARTS USED Flowers, fruit, inner bark, leaves, roots.

PHYTOCHEMICAL AND NUTRIENT CONTENT Phytochemicals: Alphaamyrin, astragalin, beta-carotene, beta-sitosterol, betulin, caffeic acid, campesterol, chlorogenic acid, cycloartenol, ferulic acid, isoquercitrin, kaempferol, lupeol, malic acid, myristic acid, oleanolic acid, p-coumaric acid, pectin, quercetin, rutin, shikimic acid, stigmasterol, ursolic acid. Nutrients: Calcium, essential fatty acids, vitamins A, B_1, B_2, B_3, and C.

ACTIONS AND USES Combats free radicals and inflammation. Relieves coughs and congestion. Builds the blood, cleanses the system, eases constipation. Enhances immune system function. Increases perspiration, lowers fever, soothes the respiratory tract, and stimulates circulation. Effective against flu viruses. The flowers are used to soothe skin irritations.

COMMENTS Also called black elder, European elder. *Caution:* Should not be used during pregnancy. The stems of this plant should be *avoided*. They contain cyanide, and can be very toxic.

Ephedra *(Ephedra sinica)*

PARTS USED Stems.

PHYTOCHEMICAL AND NUTRIENT CONTENT Phytochemicals: Beta-carotene, d-norpseudoephedrine, ellagic acid, ephedrine, gallic acid. Nutrients: Calcium, iron, magnesium, manganese, phosphorus, potassium, selenium, zinc, vitamins B_1, B_2, B_3, and C.

ACTIONS AND USES Relieves congestion, aids in the elimination of fluids, relieves bronchial spasms, and stimulates the central nervous system. May decrease appetite and elevate mood. Useful for allergies, asthma, colds, and other respiratory complaints, as well as for depression and obesity.

COMMENTS Also known as ma huang. *Caution:* Should not be used by persons who have anxiety disorders (panic attacks), glaucoma, thyroid disease, diabetes, heart disease, or high blood pressure, or who are taking monoamine oxidase (MAO) inhibitor drugs.

Eucalyptus *(Eucalyptus globulus)*

PARTS USED Bark, essential oil, leaves.

PHYTOCHEMICAL AND NUTRIENT CONTENT Phytochemicals: Alpha-pinene, beta-pinene, caffeic acid, carvone, chlorogenic acid, ellagic acid, ferulic acid, gallic acid, gentisic acid, hyperoside, 1,8-cineole, p-cymene, protocatechuic acid, quercetin, quercitrin, rutin.

ACTIONS AND USES Acts as a decongestant and mild antiseptic. Reduces swelling by helping to increase blood flow. Relaxes tired and sore muscles. Good for colds, coughs, and other respiratory disorders. Inhaling vapor from a few drops of the oil helps to break up mucus.

COMMENTS Recommended for external use only. Should not be used on broken skin or open cuts or wounds.

Eyebright (Euphrasia officinalis)

PARTS USED Entire plant, except the root.

PHYTOCHEMICAL AND NUTRIENT CONTENT Phytochemicals: Beta-carotene, caffeic acid, ferulic acid, tannins. Nutrients: Calcium, chromium, iron, magnesium, manganese, phosphorus, potassium, selenium, zinc, vitamins B_1, B_2, B_3, and C.

ACTIONS AND USES Prevents secretion of fluids and relieves discomfort from eyestrain or minor irritation. Used as an eyewash. Good for allergies, itchy and/or watery eyes, and runny nose. Combats hay fever.

False unicorn root (Chamaelirium luteum)

PARTS USED Roots.

PHYTOCHEMICAL AND NUTRIENT CONTENT Phytochemicals: Chamaelirin, helonin, saponins.

ACTIONS AND USES Balances sex hormones. Helps treat infertility, menstrual irregularities and pain, premenstrual syndrome, and prostrate disorders. May help prevent miscarriage.

COMMENTS Also called helonias.

237

Fennel (*Foeniculum vulgare*)

PARTS USED Fruit, roots, stems.

PHYTOCHEMICAL AND NUTRIENT CONTENT Phytochemicals: Alpha-pinene, benzoic acid, bergapten, beta-carotene, beta-phellandrene, beta-sitosterol, caffeic acid, camphor, cinnamic acid, cynarin, ferulic acid, fumaric acid, isopimpinellin, isoquercitrin, kaempferol, limonene, linalool, myristicin, 1,8-cineole, p-coumaric acid, pectin, protocatechuic acid, psoralen, quercetin, rutin, scopoletin, sinapic acid, stigmasterol, umbelliferone, vanillic acid, vanillin, xanthotoxin. Nutrients: Amino acids, calcium, choline, essential fatty acids, iron, magnesium, manganese, phosphorus, potassium, selenium, vitamins B_1, B_2, B_3, C, and E.

ACTIONS AND USES Used as an appetite suppressant and as an eyewash. Promotes the functioning of the kidneys, liver, and spleen, and also clears the lungs. Relieves abdominal pain, colon disorders, gas, and gastrointestinal tract spasms. Useful for acid stomach. Good after chemotherapy and/or radiation treatments for cancer.

COMMENTS The powdered plant can be used as a flea repellent.

Fenugreek (*Trigonella foenum-graecum*)

PARTS USED Seeds.

PHYTOCHEMICAL AND NUTRIENT CONTENT Phytochemicals: Beta-carotene, beta-sitosterol, coumarin, diosgenin, kaempferol, luteolin, p-coumaric acid, quercetin, rutin, saponin, trigonelline, vitexin. Nutrients: Amino acids, calcium, essential fatty acids, folate, iron, magnesium, manganese, phosphorus, potassium, selenium, zinc, vitamins B_1, B_2, B_3, and C.

ACTIONS AND USES Acts as a laxative, lubricates the intestines, and reduces fever. Helps lower cholesterol and blood sugar levels. Helps asthma and sinus problems by reducing mucus. Promotes lactation in nursing mothers. Good for the eyes and for inflammation and lung disorders.

COMMENTS Oil of fenugreek has a maple-like flavor.

Feverfew (*Chrysanthemum parthenium*)

PARTS USED Bark, dried flowers, leaves.

PHYTOCHEMICAL AND NUTRIENT CONTENT Phytochemicals: Beta-carotene, parthenolide, santamarin. Nutrients: Calcium, iron, magnesium, manganese, phosphorus, potassium, selenium, zinc, vitamins B_1, B_2, B_3, and C.

ACTIONS AND USES Combats inflammation and muscle spasms. Increases fluidity of lung and bronchial tube mucus, promotes menses, stimulates the appetite, and stimulates uterine contractions. Relieves nausea and vomiting. Good for arthritis, colitis, fever, headaches, migraine headaches, menstrual problems, muscle tension, and pain.

COMMENTS Chewing the leaves is a folk remedy, but this might cause mouth sores. Also called featherfew, featherfoil. *Caution:* Should not be used during pregnancy. People who take prescription blood-thinning medications or who regularly take over-the-counter painkillers should consult a health care provider before using feverfew, as the combination can result in internal bleeding.

239

Flax (*Linum usitatissimum*)

PARTS USED Seeds, seed oil.

PHYTOCHEMICAL AND NUTRIENT CONTENT Phytochemicals: Apigenin, beta-carotene, beta-sitosterol, campesterol, chlorogenic acid, cycloartenol, lecithin, luteolin, myristic acid, squalene, stigmasterol, vitexin. Nutrients: Amino acids, calcium, essential fatty acids, iron, magnesium, manganese, phosphorus, potassium, sulfur, vanadium, zinc, vitamins B_1, B_2, B_3, B_5, and E.

ACTIONS AND USES Promotes strong bones, nails, and teeth, as well as healthy skin. Useful for colon problems, female disorders, and inflammation.

COMMENTS The seeds are an excellent addition to a diet that is low in fiber.

Garlic *(Allium sativa)*

PARTS USED Bulb.

PHYTOCHEMICAL AND NUTRIENT CONTENT Phytochemicals: Allicin, beta-carotene, beta-sitosterol, caffeic acid, chlorogenic acid, diallyl-disulfide, ferulic acid, geraniol, kaempferol, linalool, oleanolic acid, p-coumaric acid, phloroglucinol, phytic acid, quercetin, rutin, s-allyl cysteine, saponin, sinapic acid, stigmasterol. Nutrients: Calcium, folate, iron, magnesium, manganese, phosphorus, potassium, selenium, zinc, vitamins B_1, B_2, B_3, and C.

ACTIONS AND USES Detoxifies the body and protects against infection by enhancing immune function. Lowers blood pressure and improves circulation. Lowers blood lipid levels. Helps stabilize blood sugar levels. Aids in the treatment of arteriosclerosis, arthritis, asthma, cancer, circulatory problems, colds and flu, digestive problems, heart disorders, insomnia, liver disease, sinusitis, ulcers, and yeast infections. May prevent ulcers by inhibiting growth of *Helicobacter pylori,* the ulcer-causing bacterium. Good for virtually any disease or infection.

COMMENTS Garlic contains many sulfur compounds, which give it its healing properties. Odorless garlic supplements are available. Aged garlic extract (such as Kyolic) is good. *Caution:* Not recommended for people who take anticoagulants, as garlic has blood-thinning actions.

Gentian *(Gentiana lutea)*

PARTS USED Leaves, roots.

PHYTOCHEMICAL AND NUTRIENT CONTENT Phytochemicals: Caffeic acid, carvacrol, gentiopicrin, limonene, linalool, mangiferin, sinapic acid, swertiamarin. Nutrients: Calcium, iron, magnesium, manganese, phosphorus, potassium, selenium, zinc, vitamins B_1, B_2, B_3, and C.

ACTIONS AND USES Aids digestion, stimulates appetite, and boosts circulation. Kills plasmodia (organisms that cause malaria) and worms. Good for circulatory problems and pancreatitis.

Ginger *(Zingiber officinale)*

PARTS USED Rhizomes, roots.

PHYTOCHEMICAL AND NUTRIENT CONTENT Phytochemicals: alpha-pinene, beta-carotene, beta-ionone, beta-sitosterol, caffeic acid, camphor, capsaicin, caryophyllene, chlorogenic acid, citral, curcumin, farnesol, ferulic acid, geraniol, gingerols, lecithin, 1,8-cineole, zingerone. Nutrients: Amino acids, calcium, essential fatty acids, iron, magnesium, manganese, phosphorus, potassium, selenium, zinc, vitamins B_1, B_2, B_3, B_6, and C. Ground ginger also contains vitamin A.

ACTIONS AND USES Fights inflammation, cleanses the colon, reduces spasms and cramps, and stimulates circulation. A strong antioxidant and effective antimicrobial agent for sores and wounds. Protects the liver and stomach. Useful for bowel disorders, circulatory problems, arthritis, fever, headache, hot flashes, indigestion, morning sickness, motion sickness, muscle pain, nausea, and vomiting.

COMMENTS Can cause stomach distress if taken in large quantities. *Caution:* Not recommended for people who take anticoagulants or have gallstones. Not recommended for extended use during pregnancy.

Ginkgo *(Gingko biloba)*

PARTS USED Leaves, seed.

PHYTOCHEMICAL AND NUTRIENT CONTENT Phytochemicals: Amentoflavone, apigenin, beta-carotene, bilobalide, ginkgetin, isorhamnetin, kaempferol, luteolin, myristic acid, p-coumaric acid, procyanidin, quercetin, shikimic acid, stigmasterol, tannin, thymol. Nutrients: Amino acids, calcium, iron, magnesium, manganese, phosphorus, potassium, zinc, vitamins A, B_1, B_2, B_3, B_5, and C.

ACTIONS AND USES Improves brain functioning by increasing cerebral and peripheral circulation and tissue oxygenation. Has antioxidant properties. May slow the progression of Alzheimer's disease, and may relieve leg cramps by improving circulation. Ben-

241

eficial for asthma, dementia, depression, eczema, headaches, heart and kidney disorders, memory loss, and tinnitis (ringing in the ears). Shows promise as a treatment for vascular-related impotence.

COMMENTS Can take at least 2 weeks to see results. *Caution:* People who take prescription blood-thinning medications or who regularly take over-the-counter painkillers should consult a health care provider before using ginkgo, as the combination can result in internal bleeding.

Ginseng *(Panax quinquefolius* [American ginseng], *P. ginseng* [Chinese or Korean ginseng])

PARTS USED Roots.

PHYTOCHEMICAL AND NUTRIENT CONTENT Phytochemicals: Beta-sitosterol, campesterols, caryophyllene, cinnamic acid, escin (*P. quinquefolius*), ferulic acid, fumaric acid, ginsenosides, kaempferol, oleanolic acid, panaxic acid, panaxin, saponin, stigmasterol, vanillic acid. Nutrients: Calcium, choline, fiber, folate, iron, magnesium, manganese, phosphorus, potassium, silicon, zinc, vitamins B_1, B_2, B_3, B_5, and C.

ACTIONS AND USES Strengthens the adrenal and reproductive glands. Enhances immune function, promotes lung functioning, and stimulates the appetite. Useful for bronchitis, circulatory problems, diabetes, infertility, lack of energy, and stress; to ease withdrawal from cocaine; and to protect against the effects of radiation exposure. Used by athletes for overall body strengthening. May help improve drug- or alcohol-induced liver dysfunction in older adults.

COMMENTS Siberian ginseng (*Eleutherococcus senticosus*) belongs to a different botanical family than American and Korean ginseng, but its properties are similar, and all are commonly referred to simply as ginseng. *Caution:* Should not be used by people with hypoglycemia, high blood pressure, heart disorders, asthma, or insomnia. Should not be used by pregnant women or nursing mothers.

Goldenseal (*Hydrastis canadensis*)

PARTS USED Rhizomes, roots.

PHYTOCHEMICAL AND NUTRIENT CONTENT Phytochemicals: Berberine, beta-carotene, canadine, chlorogenic acid. Nutrients: Calcium, iron, magnesium, manganese, phosphorus, potassium, selenium, zinc, vitamins B_1, B_2, B_3, and C.

ACTIONS AND USES Fights infection and inflammation. Cleanses the body. Increases the effectiveness of insulin and strengthens the immune system, colon, liver, pancreas, spleen, and lymphatic and respiratory systems. Improves digestion, regulates menses, decreases uterine bleeding, reduces blood pressure, and stimulates the central nervous system. Good for allergies, ulcers, and disorders affecting the bladder, prostate, stomach, or vagina. Used at the first sign of possible symptoms, can stop a cold, flu, or sore throat from developing.

COMMENTS Alternating with echinacea or other herbs is recommended. Alcohol-free extract is the best form. *Caution:* Should not be used by pregnant women, nursing mothers, or people with high blood pressure or insomnia. Should not be used for prolonged periods.

243

Gotu kola (*Centella asiatica*)

PARTS USED Nuts, roots, seeds.

PHYTOCHEMICAL AND NUTRIENT CONTENT Phytochemicals: Beta-carotene, beta-sitosterol, campesterol, camphor, kaempferol, saponin, stigmasterol. Nutrients: Calcium, iron, magnesium, manganese, phosphorus, potassium, selenium, zinc, vitamins B_1, B_2, B_3, and C.

ACTIONS AND USES Helps eliminate excess fluids, decreases fatigue and depression, increases sex drive, shrinks tissues, and stimulates the central nervous system. May neutralize blood acids and lower body temperature. Promotes wound healing, and is good for varicose veins and for heart and liver function. Useful for cardiovascular and circulatory disorders, fatigue, connective tissue disorders, kidney stones, poor appetite, and sleep disorders.

COMMENTS May cause dermatitis if applied topically.

Gravel root (*Eupatorium purpureum*)

PARTS USED Flowers, root.

PHYTOCHEMICAL AND NUTRIENT CONTENT Phytochemicals: Euparin, eupatorin, resin.

ACTIONS AND USES Acts as a diuretic and urinary tract tonic. Combats prostate disorders, kidney stones, and problems related to fluid retention.

COMMENTS Also called joe-pye weed, queen-of-the-meadow.

Green tea (*Camellia sinensis*)

PARTS USED Leaves.

PHYTOCHEMICAL AND NUTRIENT CONTENT Phytochemicals: Apigenin, astragalin, benzaldehyde, beta-carotene, beta-ionone, beta-sitosterol, caffeic acid, caffeine, carvacrol, catechins, chlorogenic acid, cinnamic acid, cryptoxanthin, epicatechin, epigallocatechin, eugenol, farnesol, gallic acid, geraniol, hyperoside, indole, isoquercitrin, kaempferol, lutein, lycopene, myrcene, myricetin, myristic acid, naringenin, polyphenols, procyanidins, quercetin, quercitrin, rutin, salicylic acid, tannic acid, thymol, vitexin, zeaxanthin. Nutrients: Amino acids, calcium, iron, magnesium, manganese, phosphorus, potassium, zinc, vitamins B_1, B_2, B_3, B_5, and C.

ACTIONS AND USES Acts as an antioxidant and helps to protect against cancer. Lowers cholesterol levels, reduces the clotting tendency of the blood, stimulates the immune system, fights tooth decay, helps regulate blood sugar and insulin levels, combats mental fatigue, and may delay the onset of atherosclerosis. Good for asthma. Shows promise as a weight-loss aid. May help prevent enlarged prostate.

COMMENTS To get green tea's antioxidant benefits, drink it without milk (milk may bind with the beneficial compounds, making them unavailable to the body). *Caution:* Contains a small amount of caffeine. Should not be used in large quantities by pregnant women or nursing mothers. Persons with anxiety disorder or irregular heartbeat should limit their intake to no more than 2 cups daily.

Guarana *(Paullinia cupana)*

PARTS USED Seeds.

PHYTOCHEMICAL AND NUTRIENT CONTENT Phytochemicals: Adenine, caffeine, D-catechin, saponin, tannins, theobromine, theophylline.

ACTIONS AND USES Acts as a general tonic, stimulant, and intestinal cleanser. Increases mental alertness. Improves stamina and endurance. Reduces fatigue. Useful for headaches, urinary tract irritation, diarrhea.

COMMENTS Also called Brazilian cocoa, uabano. *Caution:* Due to guarana's caffeine content, taking more than 600 mg a day is not recommended. Not recommended for people with high blood pressure or heart conditions.

245

Hawthorn *(Crataegus laevigata)*

PARTS USED Flowers, fruit, leaves.

PHYTOCHEMICAL AND NUTRIENT CONTENT Phytochemicals: Acetylcholine, adenine, adenosine, anthocyanidins, beta-carotene, beta-sitosterol, caffeic acid, catechin, chlorogenic acid, epicatechin, esculin, hyperoside, pectin, quercitrin, rutin, ursolic acid, vitexin. Nutrients: Amino acids, calcium, choline, chromium, essential fatty acids, iron, magnesium, manganese, phosphorus, potassium, selenium, silicon, zinc, vitamins B_1, B_2, B_3, and C.

ACTIONS AND USES Dilates the coronary blood vessels, lowers blood pressure and cholesterol levels, and restores heart muscle. Decreases fat deposit levels. Increases intracellular vitamin C levels. Useful for anemia, cardiovascular and circulatory disorders, high cholesterol, and lowered immunity.

Hops *(Humulus lupulus)*

PARTS USED Flowers, fruit, leaves.

PHYTOCHEMICAL AND NUTRIENT CONTENT Phytochemicals: Alpha-pinene, alpha-terpineol, beta-carotene, beta-eudesmol, beta-sitosterol, caffeic acid, campesterol, catechin, chlorogenic acid, citral, eugenol, ferulic acid, limonene, p-cymene, piperidine, procyanidins, quercetin, tannins. Nutrients: Amino acids, calcium, chromium, magnesium, potassium, selenium, silicon, zinc, vitamins B_1, B_3, and C.

ACTIONS AND USES Relieves anxiety. Stimulates the appetite. Useful for cardiovascular disorders, hyperactivity, insomnia, nervousness, pain, restlessness, sexually transmitted diseases, shock, stress, toothaches, and ulcers.

COMMENTS Placed inside a pillowcase, aids sleep. *Caution:* Should not be used by people who take antidepressants.

Horehound *(Marrubium vulgare)*

PARTS USED Flowers, leaves.

PHYTOCHEMICAL AND NUTRIENT CONTENT Phytochemicals: Alpha-pinene, apigenin, beta-sitosterol, caffeic acid, gallic acid, limonene, luteolin, pectin, tannic acid, tannins, ursolic acid. Nutrients: B-complex vitamins, iron, potassium, vitamins A, C, and E.

ACTIONS AND USES Decreases thickness and increases fluidity of mucus in the bronchial tubes and lungs. Boosts the immune system. Useful for indigestion, loss of appetite, bloating, and hay fever, sinusitis, and other respiratory disorders.

COMMENTS *Caution:* Large doses may cause irregular heart rhythms.

Horse chestnut *(Aesculus hippocastanum)*

PARTS USED Bark, leaves, oil, seeds.

PHYTOCHEMICAL AND NUTRIENT CONTENT Phytochemicals: Allantoin, citric acid, epicatechin, escin, esculetin, esculin, fraxetin, fraxin, isoquercitrin, kaempferol, leucocyanidin, myricetin, quercetin, quercitrin, rutin, saponin, scopoletin, tannin.

ACTIONS AND USES Protects against vascular damage, makes capillary walls less porous, shields against UV radiation damage. Good for varicose veins, reducing excess tissue fluids, and easing nighttime muscle spasms in the legs. Used topically, reduces pain and swelling, and prevents bruising.

Horsetail *(Equisetum arvense)*

PARTS USED Stems.

PHYTOCHEMICAL AND NUTRIENT CONTENT Phytochemicals: Beta-carotene, beta-sitosterol, caffeic acid, campesterol, equisetonin, ferulic acid, gallic acid, isoquercitrin, isoquercitroside, kaempferol, luteolin, naringenin, p-coumaric acid, tannic acid, vanillic acid. Nutrients: Calcium, iron, magnesium, manganese, phosphorus, potassium, selenium, silicon, zinc, vitamins B_1, B_2, B_3, and C.

ACTIONS AND USES Acts as a diuretic, lessens inflammation, and reduces muscle cramps and spasms. Aids calcium absorption, which promotes healthy skin and strengthens bone, hair, nails, and teeth. Bolsters healing of broken bones and connective tissue. Strengthens the heart and lungs. Useful for the treatment of arthritis, bone diseases such as osteoporosis and rickets, bronchitis, cardiovascular disease, edema, gallbladder disorders, gout, muscle cramps, and prostate disorders. Used in poultice form to depress bleeding and accelerate healing of burns and wounds.

COMMENTS Also called bottle brush, shavegrass. If this herb is used for a prolonged period, supplemental vitamin B_1 (thiamin) should be taken, as horsetail interferes with the absorption of this vitamin.

Hydrangea *(Hydrangea arborescens)*

PARTS USED Rhizomes, roots.

PHYTOCHEMICAL AND NUTRIENT CONTENT Phytochemicals: Kaempferol, quercetin, rutin, saponin. Nutrients: Calcium, iron, magnesium, manganese, phosphorus, potassium, selenium, zinc.

ACTIONS AND USES Stimulates the kidneys and acts as a diuretic. Good for bladder infection, kidney disease, obesity, and prostate disorders. Combined with gravel root, good for kidney stones.

COMMENTS *Caution:* The leaves of this plant should *not* be consumed. They contain cyanide and can be toxic.

Hyssop *(Hyssopus officinalis)*

PARTS USED Flowers, leaves, shoots.

PHYTOCHEMICAL AND NUTRIENT CONTENT Phytochemicals: Alpha-pinene, benzaldehyde, beta-ionone, beta-sitosterol, borneol, caffeic acid, camphor, carvacrol, eugenol, ferulic acid, geraniol, hesperidin, limonene, linalool, marrubiin, oleanolic acid, 1,8-cineole, rosmarinic acid, thymol, ursolic acid. Nutrients: Choline.

ACTIONS AND USES Promotes expulsion of mucus from the respiratory tract, relieves congestion, regulates blood pressure, and dispels gas. Used externally, helpful for wound healing. Good for circulatory problems, epilepsy, fever, gout, and weight problems. Poultices made from fresh green hyssop help heal cuts.

COMMENTS *Caution:* Should not be used during pregnancy.

Irish moss *(Chondrus crispus)*

PARTS USED Entire plant.

PHYTOCHEMICAL AND NUTRIENT CONTENT Phytochemicals: Beta-carotene. Nutrients: Calcium, iron, magnesium, manganese, phosphorus, potassium, selenium, zinc, vitamins B_1, B_2, B_3, and C.

ACTIONS AND USES Acts as an expectorant and aids in the formation of stools. Good for bronchitis and many intestinal disorders. Also used in skin lotions and in hair rinses for dry hair.

Jaborandi *(Pilocarpus jaborandi)*

PARTS USED Leaves.

PHYTOCHEMICAL AND NUTRIENT CONTENT Phytochemicals: Alpha-pinene, limonene, myrcene, pilocarpine.

ACTIONS AND USES Fights inflammation and acts as a diuretic. Helps stimulate milk production and flow in nursing mothers. Beneficial for fever, colds and flu, bronchitis, colon disorders, and edema. Topically, useful for baldness and for promoting circulation in the capillaries.

COMMENTS A rainforest herb whose active compound, pilocarpine, has been used for over 120 years to relieve intraocular pressure in glaucoma.

Jatoba *(Hymenaea courbaril)*

PARTS USED Bark, leaves, fruit.

PHYTOCHEMICAL AND NUTRIENT CONTENT Phytochemicals: Beta-sitosterol, caryophyllene, delta-cadinene, epicatechin.

ACTIONS AND USES Fights inflammation, free radicals, and bacterial and fungal infection. Increases energy. Beneficial for asthma, bronchitis, bursitis, bladder infection, candida and other fungal infections, arthritis, and prostatitis.

COMMENTS A rainforest herb with a wide range of traditional uses.

Juniper *(Juniperus communis)*

PARTS USED Fruit.

PHYTOCHEMICAL AND NUTRIENT CONTENT Phytochemicals: Alpha-pinene, beta-carotene, beta-pinene, betulin, borneol, camphor, caryophyllene, catechin, farnesol, epicatechin, glycolic acid, limonene, linalool, menthol, rutin, tannins, umbelliferone. Nutrients: Calcium, chromium, iron, magnesium, manganese, phosphorus, potassium, selenium, zinc, vitamins B_1, B_2, B_3, and C.

ACTIONS AND USES Acts as a diuretic, anti-inflammatory, and decongestant. Helps regulate blood sugar levels. Helpful in treatment of asthma, bladder infection, fluid retention, gout, obesity, and prostate disorders.

COMMENTS *Caution:* May interfere with absorption of iron and other minerals when taken internally. Should not be used during pregnancy. Should not be used by persons with kidney disease.

Kava kava *(Piper methysticum)*

PARTS USED Roots.

PHYTOCHEMICAL AND NUTRIENT CONTENT Phytochemicals: Cinnamic acid, kavalactones (including kawain, dihydrokawain, methysticin, dihydromethysticin, yangonin).

ACTIONS AND USES Induces physical and mental relaxation. Acts as a diuretic, genitourinary antiseptic, and gastrointestinal tonic. Relieves muscle spasms and eases pain. Helpful for anxiety and anxiety disorders, insomnia, stress-related disorders, menopausal symptoms, and urinary tract infections.

COMMENTS Also called kava. *Caution:* Can cause drowsiness. If this occurs, discontinue use or reduce the dosage. Should not be combined with alcohol. Not recommended for persons under the age of 18, pregnant women, nursing mothers, or individuals who suffer from depression or take certain prescription drugs, especially antianxiety drugs.

Kudzu *(Pueraria lobata)*

PARTS USED Leaves, roots, shoots.

PHYTOCHEMICAL AND NUTRIENT CONTENT Phytochemicals: Daidzein, daidzin, genistein, p-coumaric acid, puerarin, quercetin. Nutrients: Calcium, iron, magnesium, phosphorus, potassium, vitamin B_2.

ACTIONS AND USES Suppresses alcohol cravings. Lowers blood pressure and relieves headache, stiff neck, vertigo, and tinnitus. Useful for treating alcoholism, colds, flu, and gastrointestinal problems.

COMMENTS In China and Japan, kudzu has been used as a food starch and medicine for centuries. The Chinese use kudzu extract to treat angina pectoris.

Lady's mantle (Achillea millefolium)

PARTS USED Entire plant, except the root.

PHYTOCHEMICAL AND NUTRIENT CONTENT Phytochemicals: Achilleine, alpha-pinene, apigenin, azulene, beta-carotene, betaine, beta-pinene, beta-sitosterol, betonicine, borneol, caffeic acid, camphor, caryophyllene, chamazulene, coumarins, eugenol, guaiazulene, isorhamnetin, limonene, luteolin, mannitol, menthol, myrcene, myristic acid, 1,8-cineole, p-cymene, quercetin, quercitrin, rutin, salicylic acid, stigmasterol, tannin, thujone. Nutrients: Amino acids, calcium, fatty acids, folate, iron, magnesium, manganese, phosphorus, potassium, selenium, zinc, vitamins B_1, B_2, B_3, and C.

ACTIONS AND USES Has anti-inflammatory, diuretic, and antiviral effects. Helps to heal mucous membranes, improve blood clotting, and increase perspiration. Helps to regulate menstruation, reduce excessive bleeding, and ease cramps. Useful for muscle spasms, fever, gastrointestinal disorders, inflammatory disorders, and viral infections. Applied topically, stops bleeding and promotes healing. Good as a douche for vaginal irritation.

COMMENTS Also called soldier's herb, yarrow. *Caution:* Interferes with absorption of iron and other minerals. Should not be used by individuals who are unusually sun sensitive. Should not be used during pregnancy.

251

Lavender (Lavandula angustifolia)

PARTS USED Flowers.

PHYTOCHEMICAL AND NUTRIENT CONTENT Phytochemicals: Alpha-pinene, beta-pinene, beta-santalene, borneol, camphor, caryophyllene, coumarin, geraniol, limonene, linalool, luteolin, 1,8-cineole, rosmarinic acid, tannin, umbelliferone, ursolic acid.

ACTIONS AND USES Relieves stress and depression. Beneficial for the skin. Good for burns, headaches, psoriasis, and other skin problems.

COMMENTS Essential oil of lavender is very popular in aromatherapy. *Caution:* Should not be used during pregnancy. Lavender oil should not be taken internally.

Lemongrass *(Cymbopogon citratus)*

PARTS USED Leaves, stems.

PHYTOCHEMICAL AND NUTRIENT CONTENT Phytochemicals: Alpha-pinene, beta-sitosterol, caryophyllene, citral, farnesol, geraniol, limonene, luteolin, myrcene, 1,8-cineole, quercetin, rutin, saponin, triacontanol. Nutrients: Calcium, iron, magnesium, manganese, phosphorus, potassium, selenium, zinc.

ACTIONS AND USES Acts as an astringent, tonic, and digestive aid. Good for the skin and nails. Useful for fever, flu, headaches, and intestinal irritations.

COMMENTS Used in perfumes and other products as a fragrance.

Licorice *(Glycyrrhiza glabra)*

PARTS USED Roots.

PHYTOCHEMICAL AND NUTRIENT CONTENT Phytochemicals: Apigenin, benzaldehyde, beta-carotene, beta-sitosterol, betaine, camphor, carvacrol, estriol, eugenol, ferulic acid, formononetin, geraniol, glabrene, glabridin, glabrol, glycyrrhetinic acid, glycyrrhizin, isoliquiritigenin, isoliquiritin, isoquercitrin, lignin, mannitol, phenol, quercetin, salicylic acid, sinapic acid, stigmasterol, thymol, umbelliferone, vitexin. Nutrients: Calcium, choline, iron, magnesium, manganese, phosphorus, potassium, selenium, silicon, zinc, vitamins B_1, B_2, B_3, and C.

ACTIONS AND USES Fights inflammation and viral, bacterial, and parasitic infection. Stimulates the production of interferon and may help inhibit replication of HIV. Cleanses the colon. Reduces muscle spasms, increases fluidity of mucus in the lungs and bronchial tubes, and promotes adrenal gland function. Has estrogen- and progesterone-like effects; may change the pitch of the voice. Helps to inhibit the formation of plaque and prevent bacteria from sticking to tooth enamel. Beneficial for allergies, asthma, chronic fatigue, depression, emphysema, enlarged prostate, fever, herpesvirus infection, hypoglycemia, glandular functions, inflammatory bowel disorders, premenstrual syndrome, menopausal symptoms, and upper respiratory infections. May prevent hepatitis C from causing liver cancer and cirrhosis and protect against atherosclerosis. Deglycyrrhizinated licorice may stimulate natural defense mechanisms that prevent the occurrence of ulcers by increasing the number of mucus-secreting cells in the digestive tract. This improves the quality of mucus, lengthens intestinal cell life, and enhances microcirculation in the gastrointestinal lining.

COMMENTS Licorice derivatives have been recommended as a standard support for ulcer sufferers in Europe. Licorice-flavored candy does not work for medicinal purposes because it is mostly made with anise, not licorice. *Caution:* Should not be used during pregnancy, nor by persons with diabetes, glaucoma, heart disease, high blood pressure, severe menstrual problems, or a history of stroke. Should not be used on a daily basis for more than seven days in a row, as this can result in high blood pressure in persons with previously normal blood pressure. Extended use can cause high blood pressure, water retention, and low potassium levels.

Maca *(Lepidium meyenii)*

PARTS USED Roots.

PHYTOCHEMICAL AND NUTRIENT CONTENT Phytochemicals: Beta-sitosterol, saponin, stigmasterol, tannins. Nutrients: Amino acids, calcium, iron, magnesium, phosphorus, vitamins B_1, B_2, B_{12}, C, and E, zinc.

ACTIONS AND USES Increases energy and supports the immune system. Good for anemia, chronic fatigue syndrome, impotence, menopausal symptoms, and menstrual problems.

COMMENTS A rainforest herb that is a member of the potato family. An important food in the diet of native Peruvians, it is rich in amino acids and high in protein.

Macela *(Achyrocline satureoides)*

PARTS USED Aerial parts.

PHYTOCHEMICAL AND NUTRIENT CONTENT Phytochemicals: Alpha-pinene, caffeic acid, caryophyllene, chlorogenic acid, coumarin, delta-cadinene, galangin, luteolin, 1,8-cineole, quercetagetin, quercetin, scoparone.

ACTIONS AND USES Acts as an anti-inflammatory, antiseptic, antiviral, and antiparasitic. Stimulates and supports the immune system. Good for gastrointestinal and respiratory disorders. Useful in treating cancer, Crohn's disease, colds and flu, diabetes, menstrual problems and menopausal symptoms, and muscle aches and spasms.

COMMENTS A rainforest herb that has been found to have potential anti-HIV properties.

254

Marshmallow *(Althaea officinalis)*

PARTS USED Flowers, leaves, roots.

PHYTOCHEMICAL AND NUTRIENT CONTENT Phytochemicals: Beta-carotene, betaine, caffeic acid, chlorogenic acid, ferulic acid, kaempferol, mucilage, paraffin, p-coumaric acid, pectin, phytosterols, quercetin, salicylic acid, scopoletin, sorbitol, tannins, vanillic acid. Nutrients: Amino acids, calcium, iron, magnesium, manganese, phosphorus, potassium, selenium, zinc, vitamins B_1, B_2, B_3, and C.

ACTIONS AND USES Aids the body in expelling excess fluid and mucus. Soothes and heals skin, mucous membranes, and other tissues, externally and internally. Good for bladder infection, digestive upsets, fluid retention, headache, intestinal disorders, kidney problems, sinusitis, and sore throat.

COMMENTS Often used as a filler in the compounding of pills.

Meadowsweet *(Filipendula ulmaria)*

PARTS USED Leaves, flower tops.

PHYTOCHEMICAL AND NUTRIENT CONTENT Phytochemicals: Anthocyanidin, avicularin, coumarin, hyperoside, methyl salicylate, quercetin, rutin, salicin, salicylic acid, vanillin.

ACTIONS AND USES Tightens tissues and promotes elimination of excess fluid. Reduces inflammation and strengthens and tones the system. Good for colds, flu, nausea, digestive disorders, muscle cramps and aches, and diarrhea.

COMMENTS The word *aspirin* is derived from an old name for this plant, *spirea*. *Caution:* Because this plant contains compounds related to aspirin, it should not be used by pregnant women, and it should not be given to children with fever due to cold, flu, measles chickenpox, or any other viral infection, as this increases the risk of Reye's syndrome, a dangerous complication that can alter or damage the liver, brain, and heart.

255

Milk thistle *(Silybum marianum)*

PARTS USED Fruit, leaves, seeds.

PHYTOCHEMICAL AND NUTRIENT CONTENT Phytochemicals: Apigenin, beta-carotene, fumaric acid, kaempferol, naringenin, quercetin, silandrin, silybin, silychristin, silydianin, silymarin, silymonin, taxifolin. Nutrients: Calcium, fatty acids, iron, magnesium, manganese, phosphorus, potassium, selenium, zinc.

ACTIONS AND USES Protects the liver from toxins and pollutants by preventing free radical damage and stimulates the production of new liver cells. Also protects the kidneys. Good for gallbladder and adrenal disorders, inflammatory bowel disorders, psoriasis, weakened immune system, and all liver disorders. Has shown anticancer effects against prostate cancer and breast cancer.

COMMENTS Also called Mary thistle, wild artichoke. Because milk thistle has poor water solubility, it is not effective as a tea. A concentrated capsule or extract form is best.

Motherwort *(Leonurus cardiaca)*

PARTS USED Leaves, flowers, stems.

PHYTOCHEMICAL AND NUTRIENT CONTENT Phytochemicals: Alpha-pinene, benzaldehyde, caryophyllene, catechin, hyperoside, isoquercitrin, limonene, linalool, marrubiin, oleanolic acid, quercetin, quercitrin, rutin, saponin, stachydrine, tannin, ursolic acid. Nutrients: Vitamin C.

ACTIONS AND USES Traditionally used to relieve childbirth pain and as a tranquilizer. Helpful for menstrual disorders, menopausal symptoms, vaginitis, thyroid and rheumatic problems. Has a tonic effect on the heart. Useful for headache, insomnia, and vertigo.

COMMENTS *Caution:* Should not be used during pregnancy (until the onset of labor), as it can stimulate uterine contractions. Not recommended for persons with clotting disorders, high blood pressure, or heart disease.

Muira puama *(Ptychopetalum olacoides)*

PARTS USED Bark, roots.

PHYTOCHEMICAL AND NUTRIENT CONTENT Phytochemicals: Beta-sitosterol, campesterol, coumarin, lupeol.

ACTIONS AND USES Helps relieve pain, acts as a mild laxative and detoxifier, and supports the heart. Has a general tonic effect and balances sex hormones. Beneficial in treating nervous system disorders, impotence, depression, stress, rheumatism, hair loss, asthma, and menopausal and menstrual problems.

COMMENTS An alcohol-based extract is believed to be the best form of this rainforest herb, as the active constituents are neither water soluble nor broken down in the digestive process.

Mullein *(Verbascum thapsus)*

PARTS USED Leaves.

PHYTOCHEMICAL AND NUTRIENT CONTENT Phytochemicals: Beta-carotene, beta-sitosterol, coumarin, hesperidin, saponins. Nutrients: Calcium, iron, magnesium, manganese, phosphorus, potassium, selenium, zinc, vitamins B_1, B_2, B_3, and C.

ACTIONS AND USES Acts as a laxative, painkiller, and sleep aid. Taken internally, aids in getting rid of warts. Clears congestion. Useful for asthma, bronchitis, difficulty breathing, earache, hay fever, and swollen glands. Used in kidney formulas to soothe inflammation.

Mustard *(Brassica nigra)*

PARTS USED Seeds.

PHYTOCHEMICAL AND NUTRIENT CONTENT Phytochemicals: Allyl isothiocyanate, caffeic acid, chlorogenic acid, ferulic acid, p-coumaric acid, protocatechuic acid, sinapic acid, vanillic acid.

ACTIONS AND USES Improves digestion and aids in the metabolism of fat. Applied externally, helpful for chest congestion, inflammation, injuries, and joint pain.

COMMENTS *Caution:* Can be irritating when applied directly to the skin. Not recommended for use on children under the age of six.

257

Myrrh *(Commiphora myrrha)*

PARTS USED Resin from stems.

PHYTOCHEMICAL AND NUTRIENT CONTENT Phytochemicals: Acetic acid, beta-sitosterol, campesterol, cinnamaldehyde, cuminaldehyde, dipentene, eugenol, limonene, m-cresol.

ACTIONS AND USES Acts as an antiseptic, disinfectant, expectorant, and deodorizer. Stimulates the immune system and gastric secretions. Tones and stimulates mucous tissue. Helps to fight harmful bacteria in the mouth. Good for bad breath, periodontal disease, skin disorders, asthma, bronchitis, colds, flu, sinusitis, sore throat, herpes simplex, and ulcers. Topically, useful for abscesses, boils, sores, and wounds.

COMMENTS Used in many perfumes and in incense for its aromatic properties. Guggul, the standardized extract of the Indian mukul myrrh tree, lowers both cholesterol and triglyceride levels.

Nettle *(Urtica dioica)*

PARTS USED Flowers, leaves, roots.

PHYTOCHEMICAL AND NUTRIENT CONTENT Phytochemicals: Acetic acid, beta-carotene, betaine, caffeic acid, ferulic acid, lecithin, lycopene, p-coumaric acid, scopoletin. Nutrients: Calcium, copper, fatty acids, folate, iron, magnesium, manganese, phosphorus, potassium, selenium, sulfur, zinc, vitamins B_1, B_2, B_3, B_5, C, and E.

ACTIONS AND USES Acts as a diuretic, expectorant, pain reliever, and tonic. Good for benign prostatic hyperplasia, anemia, arthritis, rheumatism, hay fever, and other allergic disorders, kidney problems, and malabsorption syndrome. Improves goiter, inflammatory conditions, and mucous conditions of the lungs. Used in hair care products, helps stimulate hair follicles and regulate scalp oil buildup.

COMMENTS Also called stinging nettle.

Oat straw *(Avena sativa)*

PARTS USED Whole plant.

PHYTOCHEMICAL AND NUTRIENT CONTENT Phytochemicals: Benzaldehyde, beta-carotene, beta-ionone, beta-sitosterol, betaine, caffeic acid, campesterol, caryophyllene, chlorophyll, ferulic acid, lignin, limonene, p-coumaric acid, quercetin, scopoletin, sinapic acid, stigmasterol, vanillic acid, vanillin. Nutrients: Calcium, folate, iron, magnesium, manganese, phosphorus, potassium, selenium, zinc, vitamins A, B_1, B_2, B_3, B_5, B_6, and E.

ACTIONS AND USES Acts as an antidepressant and restorative nerve tonic. Increases perspiration. Helps to ease insomnia. Good for bed-wetting, depression, stress, and skin disorders.

Olive leaf *(Olea europaea)*

PARTS USED Extract from leaves.

PHYTOCHEMICAL AND NUTRIENT CONTENT Phytochemicals: Apigenin, beta-sitosterol glucoside, cinchonidine, esculetin, kaempferol, luteolin, mannitol, maslinic acid, oleanic acid, oleuropein, quercetin, rutin, tannins. Nutrients: Calcium.

ACTIONS AND USES Fights all types of bacteria, viruses, fungi, and parasites. Helps stave off colds and flu. May have antioxidant properties. Has shown potential for lowering high blood pressure. Good for virtually any infectious disease, as well as for chronic fatigue syndrome, diarrheal diseases, inflammatory arthritis, and psoriasis.

Oregon grape *(Mahonia aquifolia)*

PARTS USED Roots.

PHYTOCHEMICAL AND NUTRIENT CONTENT Berberine, tannins.

ACTIONS AND USES Purifies the blood and cleanses the liver. Acts as a laxative. Good for many skin conditions, from acne to psoriasis.

COMMENTS Has actions similar to those of goldenseal and barberry.

259

Papaya *(Carica papaya)*

PARTS USED Fruit, leaves.

PHYTOCHEMICAL AND NUTRIENT CONTENT Phytochemicals: Benzaldehyde, beta-carotene, caryophyllene, linalool, lycopene, malic acid, methyl salicylate, myristic acid, papain, phytofluene, zeaxanthin. Nutrients: Calcium, iron, magnesium, manganese, phosphorus, potassium, zinc, vitamins B_1, B_2, B_3, B_5, and C.

ACTIONS AND USES Stimulates the appetite and aids digestion. Good for heartburn, indigestion, and inflammatory bowel disorders.

COMMENTS The leaves can be used to tenderize meat.

Parsley *(Petroselinum crispum)*

PARTS USED Fruit, leaves, roots, stems.

PHYTOCHEMICAL AND NUTRIENT CONTENT Phytochemicals: Alpha-pinene, apigenin, apiole, benzaldehyde, bergapten, beta-carotene, caffeic acid, chlorogenic acid, geraniol, glycolic acid, kaempferol, limonene, linalool, lutein, myristic acid, myristicin, naringenin, p-coumaric acid, psoralen, quercetin, rosmarinic acid, rutin, xanthotoxin. Nutrients: Calcium, folate, iron, magnesium, manganese, phosphorus, potassium, selenium, zinc, vitamins A, B_1, B_2, B_3, B_5, C, and E.

ACTIONS AND USES Contains a substance that prevents the multiplication of tumor cells. Expels worms, relieves gas, stimulates normal activity of the digestive system, and freshens breath. Helps bladder, kidney, liver, lung, stomach, and thyroid function. Good for bed-wetting, fluid retention, gas, halitosis, high blood pressure, indigestion, kidney disease, obesity, and prostate disorders.

COMMENTS Contains more vitamin C than oranges by weight.

Passionflower (Passiflora incarnata)

PARTS USED Flowers, leaves, shoots, stems.

PHYTOCHEMICAL AND NUTRIENT CONTENT Phytochemicals: Apigenin, flavonoids, harmaline, kaempferol, luteolin, maltol, quercetin, rutin, scopoletin, stigmasterol, umbelliferone, vitexin. Nutrients: Amino acids, calcium.

ACTIONS AND USES Has a gentle sedative effect and helps lower blood pressure. Helpful for anxiety, hyperactivity, insomnia, neuritis, and stress-related disorders.

COMMENTS Also called maypop. *Caution:* Should not be used during pregnancy, as it may stimulate the uterus.

Pau d'arco (Tabebuia heptaphylla)

PARTS USED Inner bark.

PHYTOCHEMICAL AND NUTRIENT CONTENT Phytochemicals: Beta-carotene, beta-sitosterol, lapachol.

ACTIONS AND USES Fights bacterial and viral infection. Cleanses the blood. Good for candidiasis, smoker's cough, warts, and all types of infection. Helpful for AIDS, allergies, cancer, cardiovascular problems, inflammatory bowel disease, rheumatism, tumors, and ulcers.

COMMENTS Also called lapacho, taheebo.

Peppermint *(Mentha piperita)*

PARTS USED Flowering tops, oil, leaves.

PHYTOCHEMICAL AND NUTRIENT CONTENT Phytochemicals: Acetic acid, alpha-carotene, alpha-pinene, azulene, beta-carotene, beta-ionone, betaine, caffeic acid, carvacrol, carvone, chlorogenic acid, coumarin, eugenol, hesperetin, limonene, linalool, luteolin, menthol, 1,8-cineole, p-coumaric acid, pectin, rosmarinic acid, rutin, tannin, thymol, vanillin. Nutrients: Calcium, choline, iron, magnesium, manganese, phosphorus, potassium, selenium, zinc, vitamins B_1, B_2, B_3, and E.

ACTIONS AND USES Increases stomach acidity, aiding digestion. Slightly anesthetizes mucous membranes and the gastrointestinal tract. Useful for chills, colic, diarrhea, headache, heart trouble, indigestion, irritable bowel syndrome, nausea, poor appetite, rheumatism, and spasms.

COMMENTS *Caution:* May interfere with iron absorption. Should not be used by nursing mothers. Do not ingest pure menthol or pure peppermint leaves.

261

Plantain *(Plantago major)*

PARTS USED Leaves.

PHYTOCHEMICAL AND NUTRIENT CONTENT Phytochemicals: Adenine, allantoin, aucubin, apigenin, benzoic acid, caffeic acid, chlorogenic acid, cinnamic acid, ferulic acid, fiber, luteolin, oleanolic acid, p-coumaric acid, salicylic acid, tannin, ursolic acid, vanillic acid. Nutrients: Potassium, vitamin A.

ACTIONS AND USES Acts as a diuretic and is soothing to the lungs and urinary tract. May slow the growth of tuberculosis bacteria. Has a healing, antibiotic, and styptic effect when used topically for sores and wounds. Useful for indigestion and heartburn. Applied in a poultice, good for bee stings and any kind of bite.

COMMENTS Young leaves are tasty and can be eaten in salads. *Caution:* Do not mistake plantain for foxglove (*Digitalis lanata*), which has a similar appearance.

Pleurisy root (*Asclepias tuberosa*)

PARTS USED Rhizome.

PHYTOCHEMICAL AND NUTRIENT CONTENT Phytochemicals: Alpha-amyrin, asclepiadin, beta-amyrin, isorhamnetin, kaempferol, lupeol, quercetin, rutin, viburnitol.

ACTIONS AND USES Reduces inflammation of the pleural membranes of the lungs, enhances secretion of healthy lung fluids, and stimulates the lymphatic system. Has antispasmodic properties. Induces sweating and aids expectoration. Beneficial for pleurisy, pneumonia, bronchitis, flu, and coughs.

COMMENTS Also called butterfly weed.

Primrose (*Oenothera biennis*)

PARTS USED Seed oil.

PHYTOCHEMICAL AND NUTRIENT CONTENT Phytochemicals: Beta-sitosterol, caffeic acid, campesterol, ellagic acid, gallic acid, kaempferol, lignin, p-coumaric acid, phytosterols, quercetin, tannin. Nutrients: Amino acids, calcium, essential fatty acids, iron, magnesium, manganese, phosphorus, potassium, vitamin E, zinc.

ACTIONS AND USES Promotes cardiovascular health. Aids in weight loss and reduces high blood pressure. Acts as a natural estrogen promoter. Helpful in treating alcoholism, arthritis, hot flashes, menstrual problems such as cramps and heavy bleeding, multiple sclerosis, and skin disorders.

COMMENTS Also called evening primrose. *Caution:* Primrose *root* should not be used during pregnancy.

Pumpkin (*Cucurbita pepo*)

PARTS USED Flesh, seed.

PHYTOCHEMICAL AND NUTRIENT CONTENT Phytochemicals: Astragalin, beta-carotene, beta-sitosterol, caffeic acid, chlorogenin, cryptoxanthin, diosgenin, ferulic acid, gitogenin, kaempferol, lutein, mannitol, myristic acid, phytosterols, quercetin, ruscogenin, salicylic acid, zeaxanthin. Nutrients: Amino acids, calcium, essential fatty acids, iron, magnesium, manganese, phosphorus, potassium, selenium, zinc, vitamins A, C, and E.

ACTIONS AND USES Useful for prostate disorders and irritable bladder.

Puncture vine *(Tribulus terrestris)*

PARTS USED Flowers, fruit, leaves, stems.

PHYTOCHEMICAL AND NUTRIENT CONTENT Phytochemicals: Astragalin, beta-sitosterol, campesterol, chlorogenin, diosgenin, gitogenin, kaempferol, quercetin, ruscogenin, rutin, stigmasterol. Nutrients: Amino acids, calcium, essential fatty acids, iron, phosphorus, potassium, vitamin C.

ACTIONS AND USES Improves sex drive. Eases menopausal symptoms. Stimulates production of and balances male and female hormones. Enhances the immune system. Helps build muscles and increase stamina and endurance. Has antifungal, antibacterial, and anti-inflammatory actions. Useful as a general tonic and revitalizer for the liver, kidneys, and urinary tract.

COMMENTS Also called caltrop.

Pygeum *(Pygeum africanum)*

PARTS USED Bark.

PHYTOCHEMICAL AND NUTRIENT CONTENT Phytochemicals: Beta-sitosterol, oleanic acid, ursolic acid.

ACTIONS AND USES Reduces inflammation and decongestion. Lowers levels of inflammatory compounds in the prostate. Effective in reducing prostate enlargement.

COMMENTS Used clinically in Europe to treat benign prostatic hyperplasia.

263

Red clover (Trifolium pratense)

PARTS USED Flowers.

PHYTOCHEMICAL AND NUTRIENT CONTENT Phytochemicals: Beta-carotene, beta-sitosterol, biochanin, caffeic acid, campesterol, chlorogenic acid, coumarin, coumestrol, daidzein, eugenol, formononetin, genistein, isorhamnetin, methyl salicylate, myricetin, p-coumaric acid, salicylic acid. Nutrients: Calcium, iron, magnesium, manganese, phosphorus, potassium, selenium, zinc, vitamins B_3, C, and E.

ACTIONS AND USES Fights infection, suppresses appetite, and purifies the blood. Has expectorant, antispasmodic, and relaxing effects. Good for bacterial infections, HIV and AIDS, coughs, bronchitis, inflamed lungs, inflammatory bowel disorders, kidney problems, liver disease, skin disorders, and weakened immune systems.

264

Red raspberry (Rubus idaeus)

PARTS USED Bark, leaves, roots.

PHYTOCHEMICAL AND NUTRIENT CONTENT Phytochemicals: Alpha-carotene, benzaldehyde, beta-carotene, beta-ionone, caffeic acid, ellagic acid, farnesol, ferulic acid, gallic acid, geraniol, lutein, tannin. Nutrients: Calcium, iron, magnesium, manganese, phosphorus, potassium, selenium, silicon, zinc, vitamins B_1, B_2, B_3, C, and E.

ACTIONS AND USES Reduces menstrual bleeding, relaxes uterine and intestinal spasms, and strengthens uterine walls. Promotes healthy nails, bones, teeth, and skin. Good for diarrhea and for female disorders such as morning sickness, hot flashes, and menstrual cramps. Also heals canker sores. Combined with peppermint, good for morning sickness.

Rhubarb (Rheum rhabarbarum)

PARTS USED Roots, stalks.

PHYTOCHEMICAL AND NUTRIENT CONTENT Phytochemicals: Acetic acid, beta-carotene, caffeic acid, chrysophanol, emodin, epicatechin, ferulic acid, fumaric acid, gallic acid, isoquercitrin, lutein, p-coumaric acid, protocatechuic acid, rutin, sinapic acid, vanillic acid. Nutrients: Calcium, iron, magnesium, manganese, phosphorus, potassium, selenium, sulfur, zinc, vitamins B_1, B_2, B_3, B_5, C, and E.

ACTIONS AND USES Fights infection and eliminates worms. Enhances gallbladder function and promotes healing of duodenal ulcers. Good for constipation, malabsorption, and disorders of the colon, spleen, and liver.

COMMENTS *Caution:* Should not be used during pregnancy.

Rose *(Rosa canina)*

PARTS USED Fruit (hips).

PHYTOCHEMICAL AND NUTRIENT CONTENT Phytochemicals: Beta-carotene, betulin, catechin, epicatechin, flavonoids, isoquercitrin, lycopene, malic acid, pectin, tannin, vanillin, zeaxanthin. Nutrients: Calcium, iron, magnesium, manganese, phosphorus, potassium, selenium, zinc, vitamins B_1, B_2, B_3, C, and E.

ACTIONS AND USES Good for bladder problems and all infections. A good source of vitamin C when used fresh. Rose hip tea is good for diarrhea.

COMMENTS Many vitamin and other supplements are derived from rose hips.

Rosemary *(Rosmarinus officinalis)*

PARTS USED Leaves.

PHYTOCHEMICAL AND NUTRIENT CONTENT Phytochemicals: Alpha-pinene, apigenin, beta-carotene, beta-sitosterol, betulinic acid, borneol, caffeic acid, camphor, carnosol, carvacrol, carvone, caryophyllene, chlorogenic acid, diosmin, genkwanin, geraniol, hesperidin, limonene, linalool, luteolin, oleanolic acid, 1,8-cineole, phytosterols, rosmanol, rosmarinic acid, salicylates, squalene, tannin, thymol, ursolic acid. Nutrients: Calcium, iron, magnesium, manganese, phosphorus, potassium, zinc, vitamins B_1, B_3, and C.

ACTIONS AND USES Fights free radicals, inflammation, bacteria, and fungi. Relaxes the stomach, stimulates circulation and digestion, and acts as an astringent and decongestant. Improves circulation to the brain. Also helps detoxify the liver, and has anticancer and antitumor properties. Good for headaches, high and low blood pressure, circulatory problems, and menstrual cramps. Can be used as an antiseptic gargle.

COMMENTS Makes a good food preservative. *Caution:* Should not be used during pregnancy.

Sage *(Salvia officinalis)*

PARTS USED Leaves.

PHYTOCHEMICAL AND NUTRIENT CONTENT Phytochemicals: Alpha-amyrin, alpha-pinene, alpha-terpineol, apigenin, beta-carotene, beta-sitosterol, betulin, borneol, caffeic acid, campesterol, camphene, camphor, carnosolic acid, caryophyllene, catechin, chlorogenic acid, citral, farnesol, ferulic acid, gallic acid, genkwanin, geraniol, hispidulin, limonene, linalool, luteolin, maslinic acid, oleanolic acid, 1,8-cineole, p-coumaric acid, pinene, rosmarinic acid, saponin, stigmasterol, tannins, terpineol, thymol, ursolic acid, vanillic acid. Nutrients: Boron, calcium, iron, magnesium, manganese, phosphorus, potassium, selenium, zinc, vitamins B_1, B_2, B_3, B_5, and C.

ACTIONS AND USES Stimulates the central nervous system and digestive tract, and has estrogenic effects on the body. Reduces sweating and salivation. Good for hot flashes and other symptoms of estrogen deficiency, whether in menopause or following hysterectomy. Beneficial for disorders affecting the mouth and throat, such as tonsillitis. In tea form, can be used as a hair rinse to promote shine (especially for dark hair) and hair growth. Also used to dry up milk when women wish to stop nursing.

COMMENTS *Caution:* Interferes with the absorption of iron and other minerals when taken internally, and decreases milk supply in nursing mothers. Should not be taken by individuals with seizure disorders. Should not be taken during pregnancy.

St. John's Wort *(Hypericum perforatum)*

PARTS USED Flowers, leaves, stems, oil.

PHYTOCHEMICAL AND NUTRIENT CONTENT Phytochemicals: Carotenoids, caryophyllene, chlorophyll, flavonoids, hyperoside, isoquercitrin, limonene, lutein, mannitol, myristic acid, phenol, phloroglucinol, phytosterols, quercetin, quercitrin, rutin, saponin, tannins. Nutrients: Vitamin C.

ACTIONS AND USES Good for depression and nerve pain. Helps control stress. In laboratory studies, protects bone marrow and intestinal mucosa from x-ray damage. Applied topically, the oil aids wound healing.

COMMENTS *Caution:* Large amounts can cause heightened sun sensitivity, especially in light-sensitive people. Should not be used by people who take prescription antidepressants or any medication that interacts with MAO inhibitors. Should be used with caution during pregnancy.

267

Sangre de grado *(Croton lechleri)*

PARTS USED Bark, resin.

PHYTOCHEMICAL AND NUTRIENT CONTENT Alpha-pinene, betaine, beta-pinene, borneol, camphene, dipentene, eugenol, gamma-terpinene, lignin, linalool, myrcene, p-cymene, tannins, taspine, vanillin.

ACTIONS AND USES Fights free radicals, inflammation, and bacterial, viral, and fungal infection. Helps heal wounds and stop bleeding. Good for respiratory and skin disorders, mouth and skin ulcers, sore throat, colds and flu, candida, psoriasis, herpes, and vaginitis.

COMMENTS A rainforest herb whose name means "dragon's blood."

Sarsaparilla *(Smilax species)*

PARTS USED Roots, rhizomes.

PHYTOCHEMICAL AND NUTRIENT CONTENT Phytochemicals: Beta-sitosterol, saponin, stigmasterol. Nutrients: Iron, magnesium, manganese, phosphorus, potassium, selenium, zinc.

ACTIONS AND USES Promotes excretion of fluids, increases energy, protects against harm from radiation exposure, and regulates hormones. Useful for frigidity, hives, impotence, infertility, nervous system disorders, premenstrual syndrome, psoriasis, rheumatoid arthritis, and disorders caused by blood impurities.

COMMENTS Also called Chinese root, small spikenard.

Saw palmetto *(Serenoa repens)*

PARTS USED Berries, seeds.

268

PHYTOCHEMICAL AND NUTRIENT CONTENT Phytochemicals: Beta-carotene, beta-sitosterol, ferulic acid, mannitol, myristic acid, tannins, vanillic acid, vanillin.

ACTIONS AND USES Acts as a diuretic, urinary antiseptic, and appetite stimulant. Inhibits production of dihydrotestosterone, a form of testosterone that contributes to enlargement of the prostate. May also enhance sexual functioning and sexual desire.

COMMENTS Used clinically in Europe to treat benign prostate hyperplasia (BPH). Can be combined with nettle root for BPH also.

Skullcap *(Scutellaria laterfolia)*

PARTS USED Leaves, shoots.

PHYTOCHEMICAL AND NUTRIENT CONTENT Phytochemicals: Beta-carotene, lignin, tannins. Nutrients: Calcium, iron, magnesium, manganese, phosphorus, potassium, selenium, zinc, vitamins B_1, B_2, B_3, and C.

ACTIONS AND USES Aids sleep, improves circulation, and strengthens the heart muscle. Relieves muscle cramps, pain, spasms, and stress. Good for anxiety, fatigue, cardiovascular disease, headache, hyperactivity, nervous disorders, and rheumatism. Useful in treating barbiturate addiction and drug withdrawal.

COMMENTS *Caution:* Should not be given to children under 6.

Slippery elm (*Ulmus rubra*)

PARTS USED Inner bark.

PHYTOCHEMICAL AND NUTRIENT CONTENT Phytochemicals: Beta-carotene, campesterol, mucilage, starch, tannin. Nutrients: Calcium, iron, magnesium, manganese, phosphorus, potassium, selenium, zinc, vitamins B_1, B_2, B_3, and C.

ACTIONS AND USES Soothes inflamed mucous membranes of the bowels, stomach, and urinary tract. Good for diarrhea and ulcers and for treatment of colds, flu, and sore throat. Beneficial for Crohn's disease, ulcerative colitis, diverticulosis, diverticulitis, and gastritis.

COMMENTS Also called moose elm, red elm.

Squawvine (*Mitchella repens*)

PARTS USED Leaves, stems.

PHYTOCHEMICAL AND NUTRIENT CONTENT Phytochemicals: Alkaloids, glycosides, mucilage, saponins, tannins.

ACTIONS AND USES Relieves pelvic congestion and soothes the nervous system. Good for menstrual cramps and preparation for childbirth.

COMMENTS Also called partridgeberry.

Stone root (*Collinsonia canadensis*)

PARTS USED Whole plant, fresh root.

PHYTOCHEMICAL AND NUTRIENT CONTENT Phytochemicals: Alpha-pinene, caffeic acid, caryophyllene, limonene. Nutrients: Magnesium.

ACTIONS AND USES Acts as a diuretic, sedative, antispasmodic, astringent, and tonic. Good for the urinary tract. Breaks up mucus. Helpful for bronchitis, headache, cramps, indigestion, and hemorrhoids.

Suma *(Pfaffia paniculata)*

PARTS USED Bark, berries, leaves, roots.

PHYTOCHEMICAL AND NUTRIENT CONTENT Phytochemicals: Beta-sitosterol, saponin, stigmasterol. Nutrients: Iron, magnesium, zinc, vitamins A, B_1, B_2, B_5, E, and K.

ACTIONS AND USES Fights inflammation, boosts the immune system, and combats anemia, fatigue, and stress. Good for AIDS, arthritis, cancer, liver disease, menopausal symptoms, high blood pressure, Epstein-Barr virus and weakened immune system.

COMMENTS Also known as Brazilian ginseng.

Tea tree *(Melaleuca alternifolia)*

PARTS USED Essential oil.

PHYTOCHEMICAL AND NUTRIENT CONTENT Phytochemicals: Alpha-pinene, alpha-terpineol, aromadendrene, beta-pinene, camphor, caryophyllene, limonene, linalool, 1,8-cineole, p-cymene, terpinenes, terpinolene.

ACTIONS AND USES Used topically, disinfects wounds and heals virtually all skin conditions, including acne, athlete's foot, boils, cuts and scrapes, earache, fungal infections, hair and scalp problems, herpes outbreaks, insect and spider bites, scabies, and warts. Added to water, can be used as a douche for vaginitis and a gargle for colds, sore throats, and mouth sores (do not swallow it, however).

COMMENTS *Caution:* Should not be taken internally; can be toxic. If irritation occurs, discontinue use or dilute with distilled water, vegetable oil, primrose oil, or vitamin E oil. If irritation persists after dilution, discontinue use.

Thyme *(Thymus vulgaris)*

PARTS USED Berries, flowers, leaves.

PHYTOCHEMICAL AND NUTRIENT CONTENT Phytochemicals: Alpha-pinene, apigenin, beta-carotene, borneol, caffeic acid, camphor, caprylic acid, carvacrol, carvone, chlorogenic acid, cinnamic acid, citral, eugenol, ferulic acid, gallic acid, geraniol, kaempferol, lauric acid, limonene, linalool, luteolin, myristic acid, naringenin, oleanolic acid, p-coumaric acid, p-cymene, phytosterols, rosmarinic acid, salicylates, tannin, thymol, ursolic acid, vanillic acid. Nutrients: Amino acids, calcium, essential fatty acids, iron, magnesium, manganese, phosphorus, potassium, selenium, zinc, vitamins B_1, B_2, B_3, and C.

ACTIONS AND USES Eliminates gas and reduces fever, headache, and mucus. Has strong antiseptic properties. Lowers cholesterol levels. Good for asthma, bronchitis, croup and other respiratory problems, and for fever, headache, and liver disease. Eliminates scalp itching and flaking caused by candidiasis.

Turmeric (Curcuma longa)

PARTS USED Rhizomes.

PHYTOCHEMICAL AND NUTRIENT CONTENT Phytochemicals: Alpha-pinene, alpha-terpineol, azulene, beta-carotene, borneol, caffeic acid, caryophyllene, cinnamic acid, curcumin, eugenol, guaiacol, limonene, linalool, 1,8-cineole, p-coumaric acid, p-cymene, turmerone, vanillic acid. Nutrients: Calcium, iron, manganese, phosphorus, potassium, zinc, vitamins B_1, B_2, B_3, and C.

ACTIONS AND USES Fights free radicals, protects the liver against toxins, inhibits platelet aggregation, aids circulation, lowers cholesterol levels, and improves blood-vessel health. Has antibiotic, anticancer, and anti-inflammatory properties. Good for all arthritic conditions.

COMMENTS Used as a seasoning and the main ingredient in curry powder. Has inhibited the spread of HIV in laboratory tests. *Caution:* Extended use can result in stomach distress. Not recommended for persons with biliary tract obstruction, as curcumin stimulates bile secretion.

Uva ursi *(Arctostaphylos uva-ursi)*

PARTS USED Leaves.

PHYTOCHEMICAL AND NUTRIENT CONTENT Phytochemicals: Arbutin, beta-carotene, beta-sitosterol, ellagic acid, gallic acid, hyperin, isoquercitrin, myricetin, oleanolic acid, quercetin, quercitrin, ursolic acid. Nutrients: Calcium, iron, magnesium, manganese, phosphorus, potassium, selenium, zinc, vitamins B_1, B_2, B_3, and C.

ACTIONS AND USES Promotes excretion of fluids, fights bacteria, and strengthens heart muscle. Good for disorders of the spleen, liver, pancreas, and small intestine. Useful for bladder and kidney infections, diabetes, and prostate disorders.

COMMENTS Also called bearberry. *Caution:* Not recommended for women who are pregnant or nursing, nor for children under 12.

272

Valerian *(Valeriana officinalis)*

PARTS USED Rhizomes, roots.

PHYTOCHEMICAL AND NUTRIENT CONTENT Phytochemicals: Azulene, beta-carotene, beta-ionone, beta-sitosterol, borneol, bornyl acetate, caffeic acid, caryophyllene, chlorogenic acid, isovaleric acid, kaempferol, limonene, p-coumaric acid, quercetin, valepotriates, valerenic acid, valerenone, valeric acid. Nutrients: Calcium, choline, essential fatty acids, iron, magnesium, manganese, phosphorus, potassium, selenium, zinc, vitamins B_1, B_2, B_3, and C.

ACTIONS AND USES Acts as a sedative, improves circulation, and reduces mucus from colds. Good for anxiety, fatigue, high blood pressure, insomnia, irritable bowel syndrome, menstrual and muscle cramps, nervousness, pain, spasms, stress, and ulcers.

COMMENTS A water-soluble extract form is best. *Caution:* Should not be combined with alcohol.

Vervain *(Verbena officinalis)*

PARTS USED Flowers, leaves, shoots, stems.

PHYTOCHEMICAL AND NUTRIENT CONTENT Phytochemicals: Adenosine, aucubin, beta-carotene, caffeic acid, citral, tannin, ursolic acid, verbenalin, verbenin.

ACTIONS AND USES Strengthens the nervous system. Promotes liver and gallbladder health. Reduces tension and stress. Induces sweating. Promotes menstruation and increases mother's milk. Useful for mild depression, insomnia, headache, toothache, wounds, colds, fever.

COMMENTS *Caution:* Should not be used during pregnancy, as it stimulates uterine contractions.

White oak *(Quercus alba)*

PARTS USED Bark.

PHYTOCHEMICAL AND NUTRIENT CONTENT Phytochemicals: Beta-carotene, beta-sitosterol, catechin, gallic acid, pectin, quercetin, quercitrin, tannin. Nutrients: Calcium, iron, magnesium, manganese, phosphorus, potassium, selenium, zinc, vitamins B_1, B_2, B_3, and C.

ACTIONS AND USES Acts as an antiseptic. Good for skin wounds, bee stings, burns, diarrhea, fevers and cold, bronchitis, nosebleed, poison ivy, and varicose veins. Also good for the teeth. Can be used in enemas and douches.

White willow *(Salix alba)*

PARTS USED Bark.

PHYTOCHEMICAL AND NUTRIENT CONTENT Phytochemicals: Apigenin, beta-carotene, catechin, isoquercitrin, lignin, p-coumaric acid, quercetin, rutin, salicin, salicylic acid, tannin. Nutrients: Calcium, iron, magnesium, manganese, phosphorus, potassium, selenium, zinc, vitamins B_1, B_2, B_3, and C.

ACTIONS AND USES Relieves pain. Good for allergies, headache, backache, nerve pain, joint pain, inflammation, menstrual cramps, toothache, and injuries.

COMMENTS Contains compounds from which aspirin was derived. *Caution:* Not recommended for use during pregnancy. May interfere with absorption of iron and other minerals when taken internally. Should not be used by people who are allergic to aspirin.

Wild cherry *(Prunus serotina)*

PARTS USED Inner bark, root bark.

PHYTOCHEMICAL AND NUTRIENT CONTENT Phytochemicals: Benzaldehyde, caffeic acid, kaempferol, p-coumaric acid, quercetin, scopoletin, tannin, ursolic acid. Nutrients: Calcium, iron, magnesium, phosphorus, potassium, zinc.

ACTIONS AND USES Acts as an expectorant and mild sedative. Good for coughs, colds, bronchitis, asthma, digestive disorders, and diarrhea.

COMMENTS Also called choke cherry, wild black cherry, Virginia prune. *Caution:* Wild cherry bark should not be used during pregnancy. Also, the leaves, bark, and fruit pits contain hydrocyanic acid, which can be poisonous. A commercially prepared syrup or tincture is best.

Wild oregano *(Origanum vulgare)*

PARTS USED Leaves, shoots, stems.

PHYTOCHEMICAL AND NUTRIENT CONTENT Phytochemicals: Alpha-pinene, apigenin, beta-carotene, borneol, caffeic acid, camphor, capric acid, carvacrol, caryophyllene, catechol, chlorogenic acid, cinnamic acid, eriodictyol, eugenol, geraniol, kaempferol, limonene, linalool, luteolin, myristic acid, naringenin, naringin, oleanolic acid, 1,8-cineole, p-coumaric acid, phytosterols, quercetin, rosmarinic acid, rutin, tannins, thymol, ursolic acid, vanillic acid, vitexin. Nutrients: Calcium, essential fatty acids, iron, magnesium, manganese, phosphorus, potassium, zinc, vitamins A, B_1, B_3, and C.

ACTIONS AND USES Fights free radicals, inflammation, and bacterial, viral, and fungal infection. Boosts the immune system. Useful for acne, allergies, animal bites, arthritis, asthma, athlete's foot, bee stings, bronchitis, chronic infections, cold, cough, diarrhea, digestive problems, earache, eczema, fatigue, gum disease, headache, menstrual irregularities, muscle pain, parasitic infections, psoriasis, sinusitis, skin infections, urinary tract disorders, and wounds.

COMMENTS Oregano sold in supermarkets is usually a combination of several oregano species, and does not have the medicinal benefits of *Origanum vulgare*.

Wild yam *(Dioscorea villosa)*

PARTS USED Rhizomes, roots.

PHYTOCHEMICAL AND NUTRIENT CONTENT Phytochemicals: Beta-carotene, diosgenin. Nutrients: Calcium, chromium, iron, magnesium, manganese, phosphorus, potassium, selenium, zinc, vitamins B_1, B_2, B_3, and C.

ACTIONS AND USES Relaxes muscle spasms, reduces inflammation, and promotes perspiration. Contains compounds similar to the hormone progesterone. Good for colic, gallbladder disorders, hypoglycemia, irritable bowel syndrome, kidney stones, neuralgia, rheumatism, and female disorders, including premenstrual syndrome and menopause-related symptoms.

275

COMMENTS Many yam-based products are extracted from plants treated with fertilizers and pesticides, which may end up in the final products. The selection, cleansing, and processing of the raw materials is very important. *Caution:* Should not be used during pregnancy.

Wintergreen *(Gaultheria procumbens)*

PARTS USED Leaves, roots, stems.

PHYTOCHEMICAL AND NUTRIENT CONTENT Phytochemicals: Caffeic acid, ferulic acid, gallic acid, p-coumaric acid, methyl salicylate, tannin, vanillic acid.

ACTIONS AND USES Relieves pain and reduces inflammation. Stimulates circulation. Good for arthritis, headache, toothache, muscle pain, and rheumatic complaints.

COMMENTS Oil distilled from the leaves is used in perfumes and as a flavoring. Contains a compound composed of 90 percent methyl salicylate, a substance similar to aspirin.

Witch hazel (Hamamelis virginiana)

PARTS USED Bark, leaves, twigs.

PHYTOCHEMICAL AND NUTRIENT CONTENT Phytochemials: Beta-ionone, gallic acid, isoquercitrin, kaempferol, leucodelphinidin, myrcetin, phenol, quercetin, quercetrin, saponins, tannins.

ACTIONS AND USES Applied topically, has astringent and healing properties, and relieves itching. Good for hemorrhoids, mouth and skin inflammation, and phlebitis. Very useful in skin care.

Wood betony (Stachys officinalis)

PARTS USED Leaves.

PHYTOCHEMICAL AND NUTRIENT CONTENT Phytochemicals: Betaine, caffeic acid, chlorogenic acid, rosmarinic acid, stachydrine, tannin. Nutrients: Choline, magnesium, manganese, phosphorus.

ACTIONS AND USES Stimulates the heart and relaxes muscles. Improves digestion and appreciation of food. Good for cardiovascular disorders, hyperactivity, nerve pain, headaches, and anxiety attacks.

COMMENTS Also called betony. *Caution:* Should not be used during pregnancy.

Wormwood (Artemisia absinthium)

PARTS USED Leaves, tops.

PHYTOCHEMICAL AND NUTRIENT CONTENT Phytochemicals: Beta-carotene, chamazulene, chlorogenic acid, isoquercitrin, p-coumaric acid, rutin, salicylic acid, tannins, vanillic acid. Nutrients: Vitamin C.

ACTIONS AND USES Acts as a mild sedative, eliminates worms, increases stomach acidity, and lowers fever. Useful for loss of appetite and liver, gallbladder, gastric, and vascular disorders, including migraine. Applied topically, good for healing wounds, skin ulcers and blemishes, and insect bites.

COMMENTS Often used with black walnut for removal of parasites. *Caution:* Should not be used during pregnancy, as it can cause spontaneous abortion. Can be habit-forming with long-term use.

Yellow dock *(Rumex crispus)*

PARTS USED Roots.

PHYTOCHEMICAL AND NUTRIENT CONTENT Phytochemicals: Beta-carotene, hyperoside, quercetin, quercitrin, rutin, tannin. Nutrients: Calcium, iron, magnesium, manganese, phosphorus, potassium, selenium, zinc, vitamins B_1, B_2, B_3, and C.

ACTIONS AND USES Acts as a blood purifier and cleanser, and as a general tonic. Improves colon and liver function. Good for inflammation of the nasal passages and respiratory tract, anemia, liver disease, and skin disorders such as eczema, hives, psoriasis, and rashes. Combined with sarsaparilla, makes a tea for chronic skin disorders.

COMMENTS Also called curled dock. *Caution:* Yellow dock leaves should not be consumed in soups or salads. They are high in oxalates and may cause oxalic acid poisoning.

Yerba maté *(Ilex paraguariensis)*

PARTS USED Leaves.

PHYTOCHEMICAL AND NUTRIENT CONTENT Phytochemicals: Caffeine, chlorogenic acid, chlorophyll, rutin, tannin, theobromine, theophylline, ursolic acid, vanillin. Nutrients: Choline, inositol, nicotinic acid, pyridoxine, trace minerals, vitamins B_3, B_5, B_6, C, and E.

ACTIONS AND USES Fights free radicals, cleanses the blood, and suppresses appetite. Fights aging, stimulates the mind, stimulates the production of cortisone, and tones the nervous system. Enhances the healing powers of other herbs. Useful for allergies, constipation, and inflammatory bowel disorders.

COMMENTS Also called maté, Paraguay tea, South American holly. *Caution:* Should not be used by people who suffer from insomnia.

Yohimbe *(Pausinystalia yohimbe)*

PARTS USED Bark.

PHYTOCHEMICAL AND NUTRIENT CONTENT Phytochemicals: Ajmaline, corynantheine, corynanthine, tannin, yohimbine.

ACTIONS AND USES Increases libido and blood flow to erectile tissue. May increase testosterone levels.

COMMENTS Yohimbine, a key component of this herb, is sold as a prescription medication. *Caution:* May induce anxiety, panic attacks, and hallucinations in some individuals. May also cause elevated blood pressure and heart rate, headache, dizziness, and skin flushing. Should not be used by women or by anyone with high blood pressure; heart, kidney, or liver disease; or a psychological disorder. Should not be combined with foods rich in tyramine, such as cheese, red wine, and liver, as this may increase blood pressure to dangerous levels.

Yucca *(Yucca baccata)*

PARTS USED Roots.

PHYTOCHEMICAL AND NUTRIENT CONTENT Phytochemicals: Beta-carotene, sarsapogenin, tannin. Nutrients: Calcium, iron, magnesium, manganese, phosphorus, potassium, selenium, zinc, vitamins B_1, B_2, B_3, and C.

ACTIONS AND USES Purifies the blood. Beneficial in treating arthritis, osteoporosis, and inflammatory disorders.

COMMENTS Routinely prescribed for arthritis in some clinics. Can be cut up, added to water (1 cup of yucca in 2 cups of water), and used as a soap or shampoo substitute. Can be added to shampoo also.

INDEX

ABOUT THE AUTHORS

PHYLLIS BALCH IS a certified nutritional consultant who received her certification from the American Association of Nutritional Consultants, and has been a leading nutritional counselor for over two decades. She came to the field as a result of experiencing firsthand the benefits of using diet and nutrition as remedies for sickness.

In the 1970s, she and her children suffered from a number of undiagnosed (or misdiagnosed) illnesses and, although they had expert medical knowledge very close at hand, these maladies continued to disrupt their lives. Ms. Balch felt that there was something missing in the typical approach that treated the symptoms rather than the cause of illness. Her first introduction to the relationship between nutrition and well-being was through the late Paavo Airola, a well-known naturopath and writer. Ms. Balch then pursued her own intensive research into the science of nutrition and, by making radical changes in diet, was able to transform her own health and the health of her children. Convinced that nutrition was, in many cases, the answer to regaining and maintaining health, Ms. Balch opened a health food store called Good Things Naturally. In 1983, she published *Nutritional Outline for the Professional and the Wise Man*—now known as *Prescription for Nutritional Healing*—to share her knowledge with a broader audience. Now in its third edition, this book has had millions of readers in many different countries, and it has been translated into seven foreign languages.

Ms. Balch continues to share her knowledge with others, and has convinced many traditionally schooled medical practitioners to incorporate nutritional methods of restoring health into their practice. She is highly sought after as a visiting lecturer and also appears on television and radio programs throughout Canada and North America. Ms. Balch currently resides in Cape Coral, Florida, and Greenfield, Indiana.